LOW SODIUM COOKBOOK FOR CONGESTIVE HEART FAILURE

Delicious, low-salt recipes and expert insights to strengthen your heart and manage blood pressure.

Kingsley Klopp

To show our appreciation for your purchase, we're delighted to offer you these special bonuses as a heartfelt thank you.

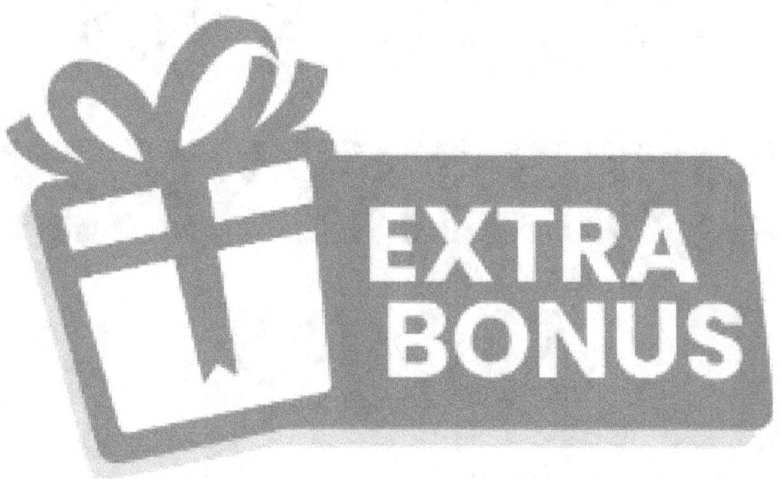

1. A Food Tracker Journal
2. Downloadable E-BOOK featuring full-color images of finished recipes

Copyright © 2024 All rights reserved.
No part of this book may be reproduced or transmitted in any form or by any means, electronic or mechanical, including photocopying, recording, or by any information storage and retrieval system, without written permission from the author. The scanning, uploading, and distribution of this book via the internet or via any other means without the permission of the author is illegal and punishable by law. The author has made every effort to ensure the accuracy of the information contained in this book. However, the author cannot be held responsible for any errors or omissions.

Table of Contents

Part 1: Understanding Congestive Heart Failure (CHF)
- What is Congestive Heart Failure?..9
- Symptoms and Diagnosis..11
- Role of Diet in Managing CHF..13

Part 2: Low Sodium Diet Basics
- What is Sodium and Why Limit It?..15
- Tips for Reducing Sodium in Your Diet...17

Breakfast Recipes
Breakfast Lentils..19
Breakfast Tacos...20
Pumpkin Spice Yogurt...21
Greek Yogurt with Nuts and Berries..22
Sweet Potato Hash..23
Mushroom and Spinach Sauté..24
Ricotta and Pear Toast..25
Cucumber Sandwich...26
Homemade Muesli Bread...27
Almond Butter on Rye...28
Cottage Cheese Pancakes..29
Whole Wheat Toast...30
 Almond Flour Pancakes...31
Buckwheat Pancakes..32
Oat Flour Waffles..33
Frittata...34
Egg Muffins...35
Barley Porridge...36
Buckwheat Porridge..37
Quinoa Porridge..38
Avocado Smoothie..39
Berry Banana Smoothie..39
Pineapple Coconut Smoothie...40

Fish & Seafood Recipes

Lemon Herb Baked Cod..41
Roasted Salmon with Dill...42
Paprika Tilapia..43
Baked Haddock with Tomatoes...44
Mustard Roasted Trout..45
Orange Glazed Halibut...46
Lemon Pepper Catfish..47
Herbed Sea Bass..48
Baked Scallops with Herbs..49
Grilled Mackerel with Lime...50
Grilled Sardines with Lemon..51
Grilled Tuna with Basil Pesto...52
Chili Lime Shrimp Skewers...53
Grilled Swordfish with Salsa Verde...54
Grilled Clams with Garlic..55
Broiled Tilapia with Thyme...56
Tom Yum Goong..57
Pan-Seared Scallops with Lemon...58
Lemon Sole Meuniere...59
Peppered Mackerel...60
Sautéed Shrimp with Ginger and Honey..61
Calamari with Lemon and Parsley...62

Poultry Recipes

Herb Roasted Chicken..63
Lemon Garlic Turkey Breast..64
Balsamic Glazed Chicken...65
Spiced Roast Turkey..66
Apple Stuffed Chicken Breast...67
 Mediterranean Turkey Meatloaf..68
Pesto Rubbed Chicken...69
Orange Roast Chicken..70
Grilled Chicken with Chimichurri..71
Turkey Burgers...72
Grilled Turkey Steaks..73
Barbecue Chicken..74
Broiled Turkey Cutlets with Dijon..75
Tandoori Chicken...76
Thai Grilled Chicken...77
Turkey and White Bean Chili..78
 Lemon Chicken Orzo Soup..79

Creamy Turkey and Wild Rice Soup..80
Chicken Piccata..81
Turkey Scallopini...82
Stir-Fried Turkey with Vegetables..83
Pan-Seared Chicken with Spinach..84
Chicken Marsala..85

Soups & Salads
Garden Vegetable Soup..86
Pumpkin Soup..87
Mixed Greens with Apple Slices...88
Beet and Goat Cheese Salad..89
Barley and Mushroom Soup..90
Split Pea Soup..91
Beetroot and Ginger Soup..92
Carrot and Coriander Soup..93
Leek and Potato Soup...94
Cauliflower Soup...95
Cabbage Soup..96
Sweet Potato and Apple Soup...97
Asian Vegetable Soup...98
Broccoli and Stilton Soup...99
Panzanella Salad..100
Endive and Orange Salad...101
Summer Corn Salad..102
Mediterranean Chickpea Salad...103
Waldorf Salad..104
Asian Slaw...105
Spinach and Strawberry Salad..106

Snacks & Desserts
Tiramisu..107
Chocolate Covered Strawberries..108
Mango Lassi...109
Orange Gelatin..110
Strawberry Shortcake...111
Fig Bars...112
Almond Joy Bites..113
Banana Bread..114
Pumpkin Pie..115
Oatmeal Cookies...116
 Cheese and Fruit Plate..117

Baked Kale Chips..118
 Frozen Yogurt Bark..119
Cucumber Sandwiches...120
Vegetable Chips..121

10-WEEK MEAL PLAN..**122**

Important Note

Congratulations on taking a proactive step towards managing your heart health with the **Low Sodium Cookbook for Congestive Heart Failur**e. This journey is about more than just reducing sodium—it's about embracing a lifestyle that supports your well-being while enjoying delicious meals.

As you explore the recipes within these pages, please keep in mind that individual dietary needs can vary significantly. What works for one person may not be ideal for another. We encourage you to adjust the recipes to suit your personal health requirements. If you find yourself unsure about any modifications or how certain ingredients might impact your condition, don't hesitate to consult your healthcare provider or a registered dietitian. They are your best allies in navigating these changes.

Additionally, while we've provided nutritional information to guide you, please remember that these values are approximate. The nutritional content may vary based on the specific ingredients and brands you choose. It's always a good idea to double-check labels and consider your unique dietary needs.

Furthermore, If our cookbook has brought joy to your kitchen and table, we'd be thrilled to hear about your experiences in an Amazon review. On the flip side, if you stumble upon any hiccups while exploring our recipes, don't hesitate to get in touch at **kloppkingsley@gmail.com.** We're here to support your cooking journey every step of the way.

Remember, this journey is about balance, not perfection. We're here to support you with recipes that make low sodium living not only manageable but truly enjoyable. Your health is our top priority, and we're thrilled to be part of your culinary adventure.

Wishing you good health and happy cooking!

Introduction

Welcome to the "**Low Sodium Cookbook for Congestive Heart Failure**"—your culinary guide to a healthier lifestyle, without sacrificing taste. Dealing with congestive heart failure can be overwhelming, but your diet doesn't have to be. Whether you're newly diagnosed or have been managing this condition for years, one thing remains crucial: reducing your sodium intake. But let's face it, when most people think of low-sodium diets, they imagine bland, boring meals. Well, that's about to change! In this book, we'll explore how to create delicious, satisfying meals that not only adhere to your dietary restrictions but also bring joy back to your dining table. You might be wondering, "How can I possibly enjoy food with less salt?" Don't worry! With a little creativity and the right ingredients, you can enhance flavors and discover new culinary favorites that make your taste buds dance.

Sodium is a sneaky ingredient found in many foods, and while our bodies need a small amount to function properly, too much can spell trouble—especially for those with heart conditions. High sodium levels can lead to fluid retention, increased blood pressure, and added stress on your heart. But by consciously reducing your sodium intake, you can help manage your symptoms and improve your overall health. When you hear "low sodium," you might picture meals stripped of all their flavor. But the truth is, it's not just about cutting out salt—it's about discovering new ways to enhance the natural flavors of your ingredients. Herbs, spices, and other seasonings will become your new best friends. Fresh garlic, rosemary, basil, and citrus can add depth and zest to your dishes, making your meals anything but dull.

In this cookbook, you'll find a collection of recipes that are anything but boring. We've gathered a variety of dishes that cater to every meal of the day—breakfast, lunch, dinner, and even snacks and desserts! From hearty soups to zesty salads, succulent entrees, and delightful treats, there's something here for everyone.
Imagine starting your day with a savory spinach and mushroom omelet, followed by a refreshing cucumber and dill salad for lunch. For dinner, how about lemon herb chicken with roasted vegetables? And let's not forget dessert—perhaps a slice of luscious, low-sodium apple crumble? These dishes not only tantalize your taste buds but also support your heart health. Think of cooking as an adventure. It's an opportunity to explore new ingredients, experiment with flavors, and take pride in preparing meals that nourish your body and soul. This cookbook will guide you step-by-step, offering tips and tricks to enhance your cooking skills and make your kitchen time enjoyable.

Managing congestive heart failure is a journey, and we're here to support you every step of the way. Each recipe is crafted with care, focusing on reducing sodium while maximizing flavor. Alongside delicious recipes, you'll find practical advice, nutritional information, and tips for making smarter choices at the grocery store.

So, are you ready to embark on this flavorful journey? The **Low Sodium Cookbook for Congestive Heart Failure** is more than just a collection of recipes; it's a lifestyle change that empowers you to take control of your health. With every dish you prepare, you're making a positive impact on your well-being and proving that delicious food doesn't need to be laden with salt. Open these pages, roll up your sleeves, and let's start cooking our way to a healthier heart. Together, we'll discover the joy of low sodium living—one delicious meal at a time. Here's to flavorful, heart-healthy cooking that brings a smile to your face and keeps your heart strong!

Part 1: Understanding Congestive Heart Failure (CHF)

What is Congestive Heart Failure?

Congestive Heart Failure (CHF) is a condition that strikes at the very core of our existence, affecting the heart's ability to pump blood efficiently. This isn't just a medical term or a diagnosis; it's a life-altering condition that brings with it a myriad of challenges, fears, and adjustments. To truly understand CHF, we need to explain what it means for those living with it, both physically and emotionally.

At its essence, CHF is a condition where the heart's ability to function as a pump is compromised. The heart, our body's vital organ, is designed to circulate blood throughout our system, delivering oxygen and nutrients to every cell and removing waste products. In heart failure, this process is impaired, leading to a cascade of effects on the body. But beyond the clinical description lies the human experience of heart failure, a journey marked by resilience, adaptation, and hope. Imagine the heart as a tireless engine, working ceaselessly to keep us alive. In CHF, this engine begins to falter. The weakening of the heart muscle means it can't pump blood as effectively as it should. This inefficiency leads to blood backing up in the veins, causing fluid to accumulate in the tissues and lungs. The term "congestive" aptly describes this buildup of fluid, which can cause swelling in the legs and ankles, and make breathing a laborious task. Living with CHF can feel like carrying a heavy burden every day. It's waking up to the realization that your body doesn't respond the way it used to, that tasks once done effortlessly now require meticulous planning and caution. It's the quiet anxiety that accompanies each short breath, the persistent fatigue that makes even the simplest activities seem daunting. But it's not just the physical toll that defines CHF; it's the emotional and psychological impact as well. For many, receiving a diagnosis of heart failure can be a moment of profound shock and fear. It's a stark reminder of our mortality, a confrontation with our own vulnerabilities. The path ahead may seem uncertain, filled with questions about longevity, quality of life, and the potential for normalcy.

However, within this adversity lies a remarkable strength. Those living with CHF often become acutely aware of the preciousness of life, of the moments that truly matter. There's a renewed focus on self-care, on making choices that support heart health and overall well-being. Diet, exercise, and medication become crucial allies in the daily battle against heart failure. Adopting a low sodium diet is one such choice, a powerful tool in managing CHF. Sodium, a mineral found in many foods, can exacerbate the symptoms of heart failure by causing the body to retain more fluid. By limiting sodium intake, individuals with CHF can help reduce fluid buildup and ease the burden on their heart. It's a lifestyle adjustment that requires dedication and discipline but offers significant rewards in terms of symptom management and quality of life.

The journey with CHF is also a testament to the importance of support networks. Family, friends, and healthcare providers become pillars of strength, offering encouragement, assistance, and expert care. It's in these relationships that those with CHF find the motivation to keep going, to face each day with courage and determination. Moreover, advances in medical research and treatment options continue to provide hope. While CHF is a chronic condition, it can be managed effectively with the right combination of lifestyle changes and medical interventions. From medications that help the heart pump more efficiently to devices that support its function, the arsenal against heart failure is continually expanding.

In the face of CHF, it's crucial to embrace a perspective of resilience and proactive management. It's about taking control where possible, making informed decisions, and seeking joy in the small victories. Whether it's a day with less fatigue, a walk without breathlessness, or a shared meal with loved ones, these moments become beacons of hope.

Hence, congestive Heart Failure is a formidable challenge, but it's also an opportunity to rediscover strength, resilience, and the profound value of life. It's a journey that, while arduous, can be navigated with the right mindset, support, and care. For those living with CHF, it's a daily testament to the enduring human spirit and the relentless pursuit of health and happiness.

Symptoms and Diagnosis

Symptoms of Congestive Heart Failure
1. Shortness of Breath (Dyspnea): One of the hallmark symptoms of CHF is shortness of breath. This can occur during physical activity, at rest, or while lying flat (orthopnea). It's caused by fluid buildup in the lungs, known as pulmonary congestion, which hampers the lungs' ability to exchange oxygen efficiently. This symptom can be particularly distressing, leading to a sense of suffocation and panic.
2. Fatigue and Weakness: The decreased pumping efficiency of the heart means that less oxygen-rich blood reaches the muscles and tissues. This results in a persistent feeling of tiredness and a significant reduction in stamina. Simple activities like walking, climbing stairs, or even getting dressed can become exhausting tasks.
3. Swelling (Edema): CHF often causes fluid retention in various parts of the body, leading to noticeable swelling, particularly in the legs, ankles, feet, and sometimes the abdomen (ascites). This swelling is due to the accumulation of excess fluid that the weakened heart can't effectively circulate.
4. Rapid or Irregular Heartbeat (Palpitations): As the heart struggles to meet the body's demands, it may beat faster or more irregularly. Patients often describe this as a fluttering or racing sensation in the chest, which can be alarming and uncomfortable.
5. Persistent Cough or Wheezing: Fluid buildup in the lungs can lead to a chronic cough or wheezing, often producing white or pink-tinged phlegm. This symptom is particularly prominent at night or when lying down.
6. Increased Need to Urinate at Night (Nocturia): The body's fluid distribution changes when lying down, causing more fluid to be processed by the kidneys at night. This results in frequent urination during sleep hours, disrupting rest and contributing to fatigue.
7. Swelling or Bloating in the Abdomen: Fluid can also accumulate in the liver and digestive tract, leading to abdominal swelling, pain, and a feeling of fullness. This can affect appetite and cause nausea or indigestion.
8. Weight Gain: Rapid weight gain can occur due to fluid retention, sometimes amounting to several pounds in a short period. This is often a sign that CHF is worsening and requires immediate medical attention.
9. Difficulty Concentrating or Decreased Alertness: Reduced blood flow to the brain can lead to cognitive difficulties, including problems with concentration, memory, and alertness. Patients may feel confused or disoriented, particularly in advanced stages of the disease.

Diagnosis of Congestive Heart Failure

Diagnosing CHF involves a combination of patient history, physical examinations, and various diagnostic tests. Early and accurate diagnosis is essential for effective management and treatment.

1. Medical History and Physical Examination: The diagnostic process begins with a thorough medical history and physical examination. Healthcare providers will inquire about symptoms, their severity, and duration. They will also check for risk factors such as high blood pressure, coronary artery disease, diabetes, and family history of heart conditions. During the physical examination, doctors look for signs of CHF, including swollen legs and feet, abnormal heart sounds, and jugular vein distention (a sign of increased pressure in the veins).
2. Electrocardiogram (ECG or EKG): An ECG records the electrical activity of the heart and can detect abnormal rhythms, heart muscle damage, and other heart-related issues. It's a quick and non-invasive test that provides crucial information about the heart's function.
3. Chest X-ray: A chest X-ray helps visualize the heart, lungs, and blood vessels. It can reveal heart enlargement, fluid in the lungs, and other abnormalities that suggest CHF.
4. Echocardiogram: An echocardiogram uses ultrasound waves to create detailed images of the heart's structure and function. It measures the size and thickness of the heart chambers, the functioning of the heart valves, and the ejection fraction (the percentage of blood the heart pumps out with each beat). This is a critical test for diagnosing CHF and determining its severity.
5. Blood Tests: Blood tests can provide valuable information about the overall health and function of the heart. Levels of certain biomarkers, such as B-type natriuretic peptide (BNP) or N-terminal pro-BNP (NT-proBNP), are often elevated in heart failure and can help confirm the diagnosis.
6. Stress Tests: Stress tests evaluate how the heart performs under physical stress, usually through exercise or medication that simulates exercise. These tests help assess the severity of CHF and its impact on physical activity.
7. Cardiac Catheterization: In some cases, doctors may recommend cardiac catheterization, a procedure that involves threading a catheter through the blood vessels to the heart. This allows direct measurement of the pressures within the heart chambers and visualization of the coronary arteries through angiography. It provides detailed information about the heart's condition and guides treatment decisions.
8. Magnetic Resonance Imaging (MRI): Cardiac MRI provides high-resolution images of the heart and surrounding structures. It's particularly useful for assessing heart muscle damage, detecting scarring, and evaluating the heart's functional parameters.

Role of Diet in Managing Congestive Heart Failure

The journey of managing Congestive Heart Failure (CHF) is one filled with daily challenges, emotional highs and lows, and the constant pursuit of better health. Among the most crucial elements in this journey is diet—what we choose to nourish our bodies with can significantly impact the progression of CHF, our overall well-being, and our quality of life.

The Heart and Food Connection
Our heart is a remarkable organ, tirelessly pumping blood throughout our bodies. When it's compromised by CHF, every decision we make can either alleviate its burden or add to it. Diet plays a central role in this equation. The foods we consume can either support heart health, reduce symptoms, and improve quality of life, or they can exacerbate the condition, leading to more severe symptoms and complications.

Sodium: The Silent Culprit
One of the most critical aspects of a heart-healthy diet for those with CHF is managing sodium intake. Sodium, while essential for various bodily functions, can be detrimental in excess, particularly for those with heart failure. High sodium levels cause the body to retain fluid, increasing the volume of blood the heart must pump and leading to fluid buildup in the lungs, legs, and other parts of the body. This can worsen symptoms like shortness of breath, swelling, and fatigue.

Reducing sodium intake is not just a dietary adjustment; it's a powerful act of self-care. It's about reading labels meticulously, choosing fresh over processed foods, and being mindful of the hidden sodium in everyday meals. It's a conscious effort to give your heart the best possible environment to heal and function optimally.

Embracing Fresh, Whole Foods
A diet rich in fresh, whole foods is a cornerstone of managing CHF. Fresh fruits and vegetables, whole grains, lean proteins, and healthy fats form the basis of a heart-friendly diet. These foods provide essential nutrients that support overall health and help reduce the strain on the heart.

Fruits and vegetables, with their abundance of vitamins, minerals, and antioxidants, help combat inflammation and oxidative stress, both of which are detrimental to heart health. Whole grains like oats, brown rice, and quinoa provide sustained energy without causing spikes in blood sugar levels, which can be harmful to the heart.

Lean proteins, such as fish, poultry, beans, and legumes, support muscle health and repair without the added burden of unhealthy fats. Incorporating healthy fats from sources like avocados, nuts, seeds, and olive oil helps maintain healthy cholesterol levels and provides long-lasting satiety.

Hydration: Balancing Act
Managing fluid intake is another crucial component of dietary management in CHF. While staying hydrated is essential for overall health, those with CHF often need to monitor and sometimes limit their fluid intake to prevent fluid overload. This delicate balance requires careful planning and attention, ensuring that the body gets enough fluids to function well without putting undue pressure on the heart.

The Emotional Journey of Dietary Changes
Adapting to a new dietary regimen can be an emotional journey. Food is deeply intertwined with our culture, traditions, and daily routines. Changing how we eat can feel like a loss, a departure from comfort foods, and favorite meals. It's normal to feel a sense of grief or frustration during this transition.

However, it's also an opportunity for discovery and growth. Exploring new recipes, learning to cook with fresh, flavorful ingredients, and finding joy in nourishing the body in healthier ways can be incredibly rewarding. It's about redefining the relationship with food, not as a source of immediate gratification but as a powerful tool for long-term health and vitality.

Support and Empowerment
Navigating dietary changes alone can be daunting. This is where support from family, friends, and healthcare providers becomes invaluable. Engaging with a dietitian or nutritionist who specializes in heart health can provide personalized guidance, practical tips, and emotional support. They can help create meal plans that are not only heart-healthy but also enjoyable and satisfying.

Family and friends play a crucial role, too. Sharing meals, cooking together, and supporting each other's dietary choices can make the journey less lonely and more empowering. It's about building a community of care where everyone is committed to the collective well-being.

Part 2: Low Sodium Diet Basics

What is Sodium and Why Limit It?

What is Sodium?
Sodium, often referred to simply as salt, is a mineral found in many foods and added to others as seasoning or preservative. Chemically, it is one of the electrolytes that helps maintain the body's fluid balance, transmit nerve signals, and support muscle function. Sodium is present naturally in foods like vegetables, dairy products, and meat, but it is most commonly consumed through table salt (sodium chloride) and processed foods.

In a healthy individual, the kidneys regulate sodium levels in the body, excreting excess amounts through urine. However, in people with CHF, the heart's impaired function can disrupt this balance, making it crucial to monitor and limit sodium intake.

The Role of Sodium in the Body
1. Fluid Balance: Sodium helps control the amount of water in and around your cells. It maintains the body's fluid balance by attracting and holding water, ensuring that blood pressure remains stable and organs function properly.
2. Nerve and Muscle Function: Sodium is essential for transmitting nerve impulses and muscle contractions. It allows nerves to send signals and muscles to contract and relax, supporting everything from heartbeat regulation to digestion.
3. Blood Pressure Regulation: Sodium influences blood volume and, consequently, blood pressure. Higher sodium levels can increase blood volume by retaining more water, leading to elevated blood pressure.

Why Limit Sodium in Congestive Heart Failure?
For individuals with CHF, the relationship between sodium and fluid retention becomes a significant concern. Here's why limiting sodium is crucial:
1. Preventing Fluid Retention: One of the primary symptoms of CHF is fluid buildup in the body, leading to swelling (edema) in the legs, ankles, feet, and sometimes the abdomen. Excess sodium exacerbates this problem by causing the body to retain more water, increasing the volume of blood the heart must pump and worsening the symptoms of CHF.
2. Reducing Blood Pressure: High sodium intake can lead to increased blood pressure, which puts additional strain on the heart. For those with CHF, managing blood pressure is vital to reduce the workload on the heart and prevent further damage.

3. Improving Heart Function: By limiting sodium, individuals with CHF can help maintain a healthier balance of fluids in their bodies, reducing the congestion and easing the strain on their heart. This can lead to improved symptoms, better quality of life, and potentially a slower progression of the disease.

4. Enhancing Medication Efficacy: Many medications used to treat CHF, such as diuretics, work by helping the body eliminate excess sodium and water. A high-sodium diet can counteract the effectiveness of these medications, making it harder to manage the condition effectively.

Emotional and Practical Support
Adjusting to a low-sodium diet can be challenging, particularly because sodium is so prevalent in many foods. This transition often requires significant changes in shopping, cooking, and eating habits. It's normal to feel overwhelmed or resistant at first, but with time and support, it becomes manageable. Seeking support from family, friends, and healthcare professionals can make a significant difference. Joining a support group or working with a dietitian can provide practical advice, encouragement, and new recipe ideas. These connections can help you stay motivated and on track, transforming a daunting lifestyle change into a shared journey toward better health.

Tips for Reducing Sodium in Your Diet

1. Understand Sodium Content and Recommended Limits

The first step in reducing sodium intake is understanding how much sodium is in the foods you eat and what the recommended daily limits are. For most adults, the American Heart Association recommends no more than 2,300 milligrams (mg) of sodium per day, with an ideal limit of 1,500 mg for those with high blood pressure, CHF, or other heart conditions.

2. Read Food Labels Carefully

Food labels provide crucial information about sodium content. Pay attention to the following:

- Serving Size: Ensure you check the serving size and calculate the total sodium content based on how much you plan to consume.
- % Daily Value (%DV): This indicates how much a serving of the food contributes to your daily sodium intake. Aim for foods with 5% DV or less per serving.
- Ingredients List: Look for words like sodium, salt, and soda, as they indicate the presence of sodium. Ingredients like monosodium glutamate (MSG), baking soda, and baking powder also add sodium.

3. Choose Fresh and Whole Foods

Fresh, unprocessed foods typically contain less sodium than processed and packaged foods. Focus on:

- Fruits and Vegetables: These are naturally low in sodium and rich in essential nutrients. Incorporate a variety of fresh or frozen (without added sauces) fruits and vegetables into your diet.
- Whole Grains: Foods like brown rice, quinoa, oats, and whole wheat products are good choices.
- Lean Proteins: Opt for fresh meats, poultry, fish, beans, and legumes. Avoid processed meats like bacon, sausages, and deli meats, which are high in sodium.

4. Cook at Home

Preparing meals at home allows you to control the ingredients and the amount of sodium added. Here are some tips:

- Use Fresh Ingredients: Cook with fresh herbs, spices, garlic, onions, lemon juice, and vinegar to add flavor without salt.
- Limit Salt in Recipes: Gradually reduce the amount of salt called for in recipes. Often, you can use half the amount or omit it entirely without compromising flavor.
- Experiment with Salt-Free Seasonings: Use salt-free seasoning blends, herbs, and spices like basil, oregano, thyme, cumin, coriander, and paprika.

5. Be Mindful of Condiments and Sauces

Condiments, sauces, and dressings can be significant sources of hidden sodium. Consider the following:

- Limit High-Sodium Condiments: Soy sauce, ketchup, mustard, and salad dressings often contain high sodium levels. Use them sparingly or choose low-sodium versions.
- Make Your Own Sauces: Prepare homemade versions of sauces and dressings using fresh ingredients. For example, blend olive oil, vinegar, and herbs for a low-sodium salad dressing.

6. Reduce Processed and Packaged Foods

Processed and packaged foods are notorious for their high sodium content. Reduce your consumption of:

- Canned Soups and Vegetables: Choose low-sodium or no-salt-added versions. Rinse canned vegetables under water to reduce sodium content.
- Snack Foods: Chips, crackers, and salted nuts are often high in sodium. Opt for unsalted or lightly salted versions, or choose fresh snacks like fruit, vegetables, and yogurt.
- Frozen Meals: These often contain high levels of sodium for preservation. If you must use frozen meals, look for those labeled "low sodium" or "reduced sodium."

7. Eat Out Wisely

Dining out can be challenging when trying to reduce sodium intake. Here are some strategies:

- Ask for Modifications: Request that your meal be prepared without added salt or ask for sauces and dressings on the side.
- Choose Wisely: Opt for grilled, baked, or steamed dishes instead of fried or breaded items. Avoid dishes with soy sauce, broth, or other high-sodium ingredients.
- Portion Control: Restaurant portions are often large and can contribute to higher sodium intake. Consider sharing a meal or taking half home for another meal.

8. Hydrate with Water

Staying hydrated with water can help your body manage sodium levels. Avoid beverages with added sodium, such as certain sports drinks and sodas. Drink plenty of water throughout the day to help flush excess sodium from your system.

9. Plan and Prepare Meals

Meal planning and preparation can help you maintain a low-sodium diet:

- Plan Weekly Menus: Plan your meals and snacks for the week, focusing on low-sodium options.
- Prepare in Bulk: Cook large batches of low-sodium meals and freeze portions for future use. This can make it easier to avoid high-sodium convenience foods.
- Healthy Snacking: Keep low-sodium snacks on hand, such as fresh fruit, unsalted nuts, and cut vegetables, to avoid the temptation of high-sodium snacks.

Breakfast Recipes

1. Breakfast Lentils
Ingredients
- 1 cup dry green or brown lentils
- 2 cups water
- 1 medium onion, finely chopped
- 2 cloves garlic, minced
- 1 medium carrot, diced
- 1 celery stalk, diced
- 1 teaspoon ground cumin
- 1 teaspoon ground coriander
- 1 teaspoon turmeric
- 1 tablespoon olive oil
- 1 cup baby spinach
- Juice of 1 lemon
- Fresh parsley for garnish

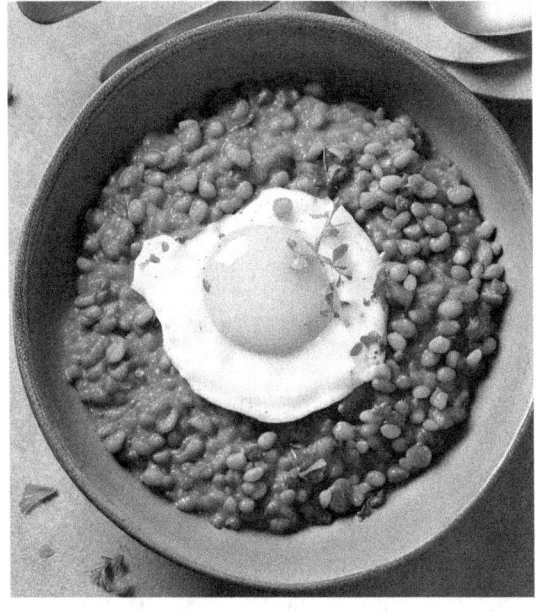

Instructions
1. Rinse lentils under cold water.
2. In a medium saucepan, combine lentils and water. Bring to a boil, then reduce heat and simmer for 20-25 minutes or until lentils are tender. Drain any excess water.
3. In a large skillet, heat olive oil over medium heat. Add onion, garlic, carrot, and celery. Cook for about 5 minutes until vegetables are tender.
4. Stir in cumin, coriander, and turmeric. Cook for another minute until fragrant.
5. Add cooked lentils to the skillet and mix well. Cook for an additional 5 minutes, stirring occasionally.
6. Stir in baby spinach until wilted.
7. Remove from heat and stir in lemon juice.
8. Garnish with fresh parsley and serve warm.

Nutrition Info per Serving
- Calories: 200 Protein: 12g Carbohydrates: 30g
- Dietary Fiber: 14g
- Sugars: 4g
- Fat: 5g
- Saturated Fat: 0.5g
- Sodium: 15mg

Serves
4 servings
Cooking Time
35 minutes

2. Breakfast Tacos

Ingredients
- 4 small whole wheat tortillas
- 4 large eggs
- 1/4 cup low-fat milk
- 1 small avocado, sliced
- 1 cup cherry tomatoes, halved
- 1/2 cup black beans, rinsed and drained
- 1/4 cup fresh cilantro, chopped
- 1 lime, cut into wedges
- 1 tablespoon olive oil
- 1/2 teaspoon paprika
- 1/2 teaspoon ground cumin

Instructions
1. In a bowl, whisk eggs with milk until well combined.
2. Heat olive oil in a non-stick skillet over medium heat.
3. Pour egg mixture into the skillet and cook, stirring gently, until scrambled and just set, about 3-5 minutes.
4. Warm tortillas in a separate pan or microwave.
5. Divide scrambled eggs among the tortillas.
6. Top each taco with avocado slices, cherry tomatoes, black beans, and cilantro.
7. Sprinkle with paprika and ground cumin.
8. Serve with lime wedges on the side.

Nutrition Info per Serving
- Calories: 250
- Protein: 12g
- Carbohydrates: 30g
- Dietary Fiber: 8g
- Sugars: 3g
- Fat: 10g
- Saturated Fat: 2g
- Sodium: 90mg

Serves
4 servings

Cooking Time
20 minutes

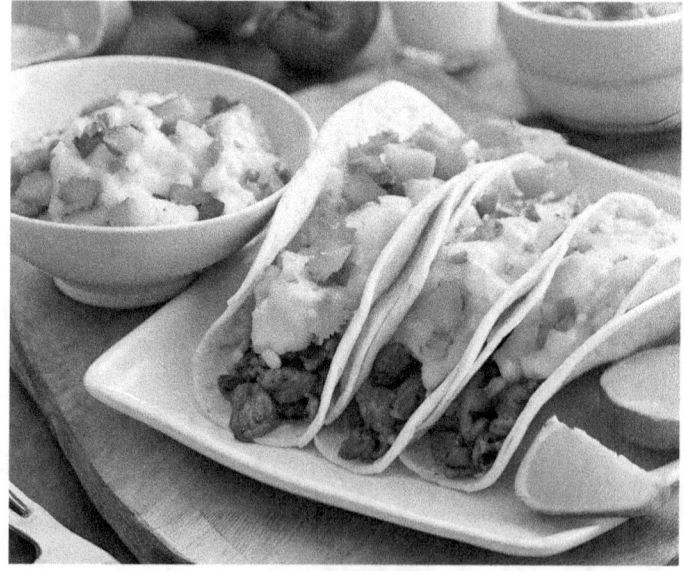

3. Pumpkin Spice Yogurt

Ingredients
- 1 cup plain Greek yogurt (low-fat)
- 1/2 cup canned pumpkin (unsweetened)
- 1 tablespoon honey
- 1/2 teaspoon ground cinnamon
- 1/4 teaspoon ground nutmeg
- 1/4 teaspoon ground ginger
- 1/4 teaspoon ground cloves
- 1/4 cup granola (low-sodium)

Instructions
1. In a bowl, combine Greek yogurt and canned pumpkin until smooth.
2. Stir in honey, cinnamon, nutmeg, ginger, and cloves.
3. Divide the mixture into two bowls.
4. Top each bowl with 2 tablespoons of granola.
5. Serve immediately or refrigerate until ready to eat.

Nutrition Info per Serving
- Calories: 180
- Protein: 10g
- Carbohydrates: 30g
- Dietary Fiber: 4g
- Sugars: 18g
- Fat: 3g
- Saturated Fat: 1g
- Sodium: 50mg

Serves
2 servings

Cooking Time
5 minutes

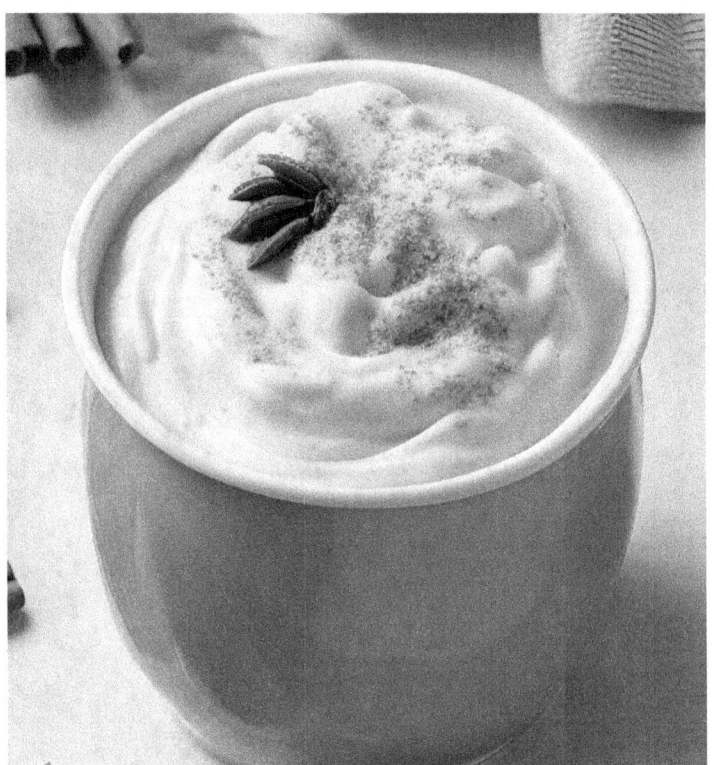

4. Greek Yogurt with Nuts and Berries

Ingredients
- 2 cups plain Greek yogurt (low-fat)
- 1 cup mixed berries (strawberries, blueberries, raspberries)
- 1/4 cup mixed nuts (unsalted almonds, walnuts, pecans), chopped
- 1 tablespoon honey
- 1 teaspoon vanilla extract

Instructions
1. In a bowl, mix Greek yogurt with honey and vanilla extract until well combined.
2. Divide the yogurt mixture into two bowls.
3. Top each bowl with mixed berries and chopped nuts.
4. Serve immediately.

Nutrition Info per Serving
- Calories: 200
- Protein: 15g
- Carbohydrates: 20g
- Dietary Fiber: 4g
- Sugars: 12g
- Fat: 8g
- Saturated Fat: 2g
- Sodium: 60mg

Serves
2 servings

Cooking Time
5 minutes

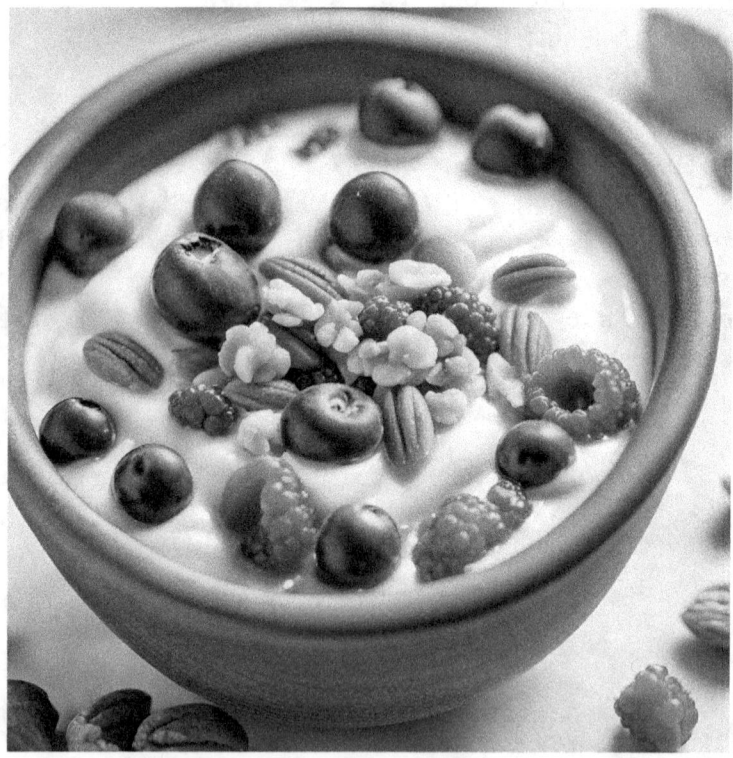

5. Sweet Potato Hash

Ingredients
- 2 medium sweet potatoes, peeled and diced
- 1 red bell pepper, diced
- 1 green bell pepper, diced
- 1 small red onion, diced
- 2 cloves garlic, minced
- 1 tablespoon olive oil
- 1 teaspoon paprika
- 1 teaspoon ground cumin
- 1 teaspoon dried thyme
- 1/4 teaspoon cayenne pepper (optional)
- Fresh parsley for garnish

Instructions
1. Heat olive oil in a large skillet over medium heat.
2. Add sweet potatoes and cook for 10-12 minutes, stirring occasionally, until they begin to soften.
3. Add bell peppers, onion, and garlic to the skillet. Cook for an additional 5-7 minutes until vegetables are tender.
4. Stir in paprika, cumin, thyme, and cayenne pepper (if using). Cook for another 2 minutes, stirring well to coat the vegetables.
5. Remove from heat and garnish with fresh parsley.
6. Serve warm.

Nutrition Info per Serving
- Calories: 150
- Protein: 2g
- Carbohydrates: 28g
- Dietary Fiber: 6g
- Sugars: 8g
- Fat: 5g
- Saturated Fat: 0.5g
- Sodium: 40mg

Serves
4 servings

Cooking Time
25 minutes

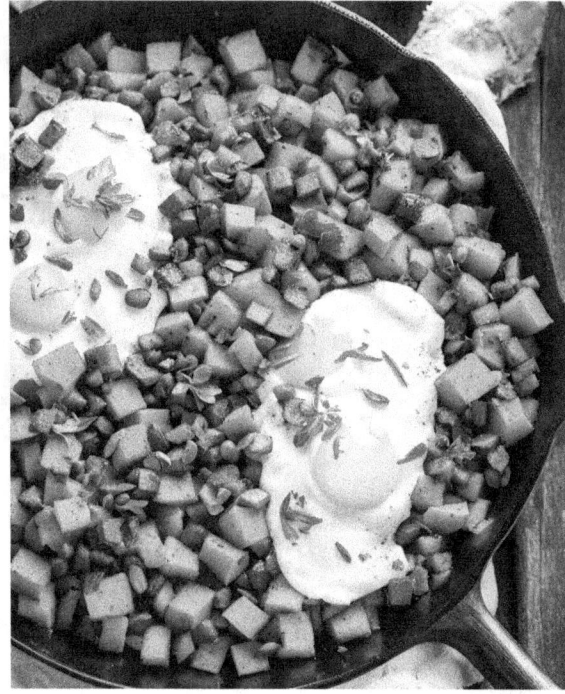

6. Mushroom and Spinach Sauté

Ingredients
- 1 tablespoon olive oil
- 1 small onion, finely chopped
- 2 cloves garlic, minced
- 2 cups mushrooms, sliced
- 4 cups fresh spinach leaves
- 1 teaspoon dried thyme
- 1 teaspoon paprika
- Juice of 1 lemon
- Fresh parsley for garnish

Instructions
1. Heat olive oil in a large skillet over medium heat.
2. Add onion and garlic, and sauté until fragrant, about 3 minutes.
3. Add mushrooms and cook until they release their moisture and begin to brown, about 5-7 minutes.
4. Stir in thyme and paprika, and cook for another minute.
5. Add spinach and cook until wilted, about 2-3 minutes.
6. Remove from heat, stir in lemon juice, and garnish with fresh parsley.
7. Serve immediately.

Nutrition Info per Serving
- Calories: 110
- Protein: 4g
- Carbohydrates: 10g
- Dietary Fiber: 4g
- Sugars: 3g
- Fat: 7g
- Saturated Fat: 1g
- Sodium: 25mg

Serves
2 servings

Cooking Time
15 minutes

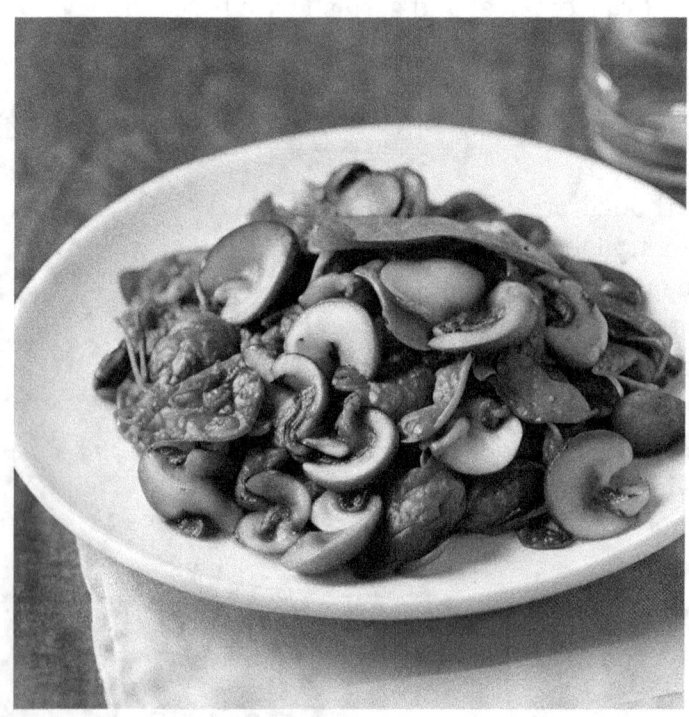

7. Ricotta and Pear Toast

Ingredients
- 4 slices whole grain bread
- 1 cup ricotta cheese (low-fat)
- 2 ripe pears, thinly sliced
- 1 tablespoon honey
- 1 teaspoon ground cinnamon

Instructions
1. Toast the bread slices until golden brown.
2. Spread a quarter cup of ricotta cheese on each slice of toast.
3. Arrange pear slices on top of the ricotta.
4. Drizzle honey over the pears.
5. Sprinkle with ground cinnamon.
6. Serve immediately.

Nutrition Info per Serving
- Calories: 250
- Protein: 10g
- Carbohydrates: 35g
- Dietary Fiber: 5g
- Sugars: 15g
- Fat: 8g
- Saturated Fat: 3g
- Sodium: 90mg

Serves
4 servings

Cooking Time
10 minutes

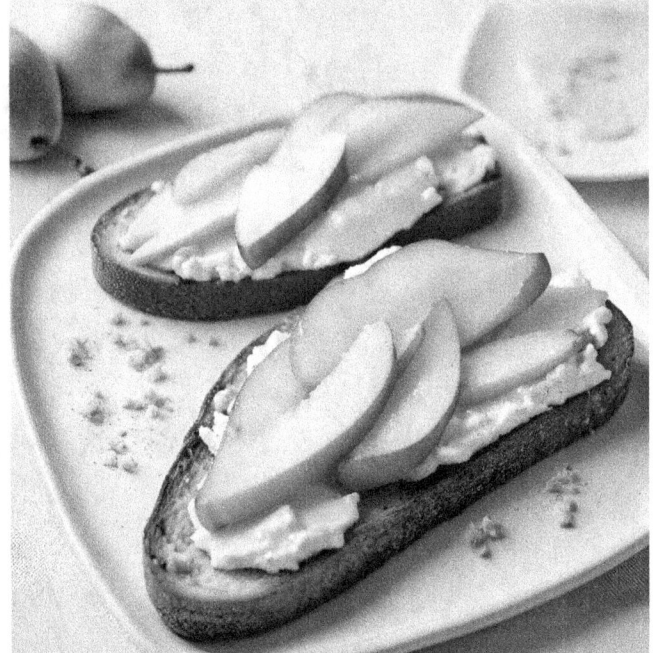

8. Cucumber Sandwich

Ingredients
- 8 slices whole grain bread
- 4 tablespoons cream cheese (low-fat)
- 1 large cucumber, thinly sliced
- 1 tablespoon fresh dill, chopped
- 1 tablespoon lemon juice

Instructions
1. Spread 1 tablespoon of cream cheese on each of the 8 slices of bread.
2. Layer cucumber slices on 4 of the bread slices.
3. Sprinkle fresh dill over the cucumber.
4. Drizzle lemon juice over the cucumber and dill.
5. Top with the remaining bread slices to form sandwiches.
6. Cut each sandwich in half and serve.

Nutrition Info per Serving
- Calories: 180
- Protein: 6g
- Carbohydrates: 30g
- Dietary Fiber: 4g
- Sugars: 4g
- Fat: 5g
- Saturated Fat: 2g
- Sodium: 120mg

Serves
4 servings

Cooking Time
10 minutes

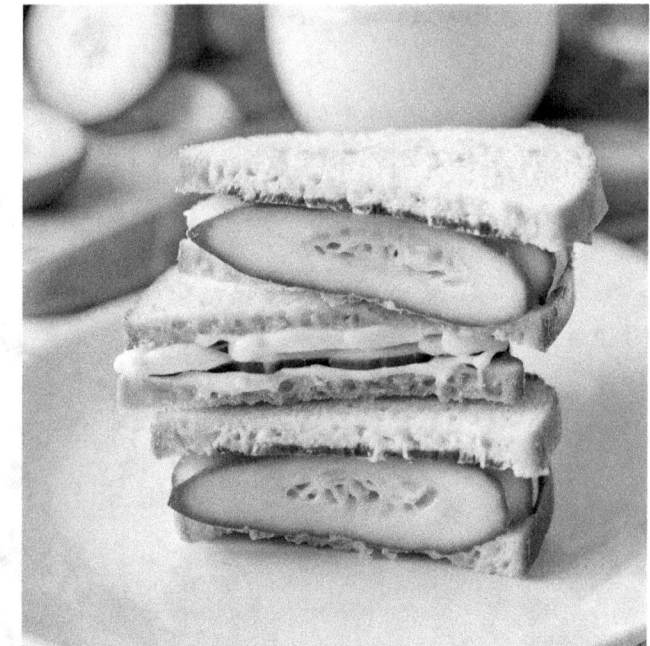

9. Homemade Muesli Bread

Ingredients
- 2 cups whole wheat flour
- 1 cup rolled oats
- 1/4 cup flaxseeds
- 1/4 cup sunflower seeds (unsalted)
- 1/4 cup raisins
- 1/4 cup chopped dried apricots
- 1/4 cup honey
- 1 1/4 cups warm water
- 2 tablespoons olive oil
- 2 teaspoons active dry yeast

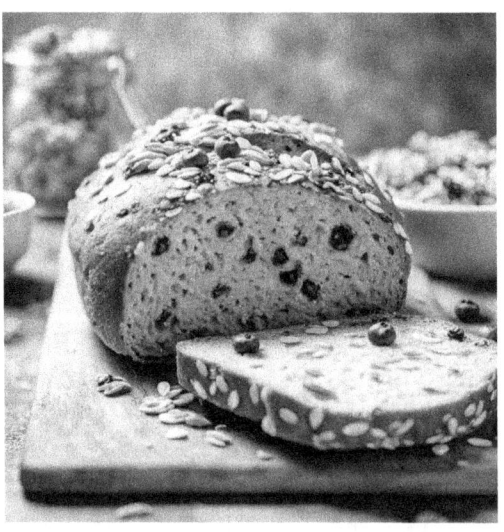

Instructions
1. Preheat oven to 350°F (175°C).
2. In a large bowl, combine whole wheat flour, rolled oats, flaxseeds, sunflower seeds, raisins, and dried apricots.
3. In a small bowl, dissolve honey in warm water. Stir in yeast and let it sit for 5 minutes until foamy.
4. Add olive oil to the yeast mixture and stir well.
5. Pour the yeast mixture into the dry ingredients and mix until a dough forms.
6. Knead the dough on a floured surface for about 5 minutes until smooth.
7. Place the dough in a lightly oiled bowl, cover, and let it rise in a warm place for 1 hour or until doubled in size.
8. Punch down the dough, shape it into a loaf, and place it in a greased loaf pan.
9. Let it rise for another 30 minutes.
10. Bake in the preheated oven for 35-40 minutes until the bread sounds hollow when tapped.
11. Allow to cool before slicing and serving.

Nutrition Info per Serving
- Calories: 200
- Protein: 5g
- Carbohydrates: 35g
- Dietary Fiber: 6g
- Sugars: 10g
- Fat: 5g
- Saturated Fat: 0.5g
- Sodium: 10mg

Serves
12 slices

Cooking Time
2 hours 30 minutes (including rising time)

10. Almond Butter on Rye

Ingredients
- 4 slices rye bread
- 4 tablespoons almond butter (unsalted)
- 1 medium banana, sliced
- 1 tablespoon chia seeds
- 1 teaspoon ground cinnamon

Instructions
1. Toast the rye bread slices until golden brown.
2. Spread 1 tablespoon of almond butter on each slice of toast.
3. Arrange banana slices on top of the almond butter.
4. Sprinkle chia seeds and ground cinnamon over the banana slices.
5. Serve immediately.

Nutrition Info per Serving
- Calories: 250
- Protein: 7g
- Carbohydrates: 35g
- Dietary Fiber: 8g
- Sugars: 10g
- Fat: 10g
- Saturated Fat: 1g
- Sodium: 80mg

Serves
4 servings
Cooking Time
5 minutes

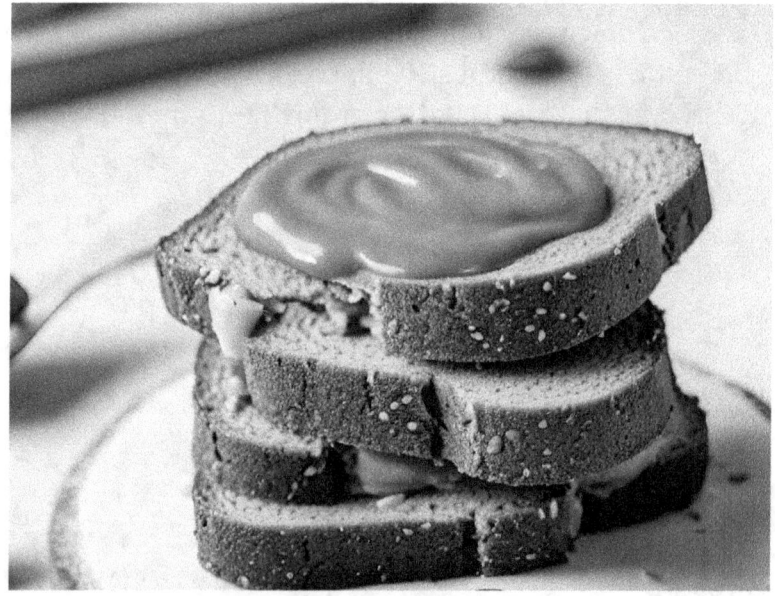

11. Cottage Cheese Pancakes

Ingredients
- 1 cup cottage cheese (low-fat, no added salt)
- 3 large eggs
- 1/2 cup whole wheat flour
- 1/4 cup rolled oats
- 1 teaspoon baking powder (low sodium)
- 1 teaspoon vanilla extract
- 1 tablespoon honey
- 1 tablespoon olive oil (for cooking)

Instructions
1. In a blender, combine cottage cheese, eggs, whole wheat flour, rolled oats, baking powder, vanilla extract, and honey. Blend until smooth.
2. Heat a non-stick skillet over medium heat and add a small amount of olive oil.
3. Pour 1/4 cup of batter onto the skillet for each pancake.
4. Cook for about 2-3 minutes on each side, until golden brown and cooked through.
5. Serve warm with fresh fruit or a drizzle of maple syrup.

Nutrition Info per Serving
- Calories: 140
- Protein: 10g
- Carbohydrates: 15g
- Dietary Fiber: 2g
- Sugars: 5g
- Fat: 5g
- Saturated Fat: 1g
- Sodium: 140mg

Serves
4 servings
Cooking Time
20 minutes

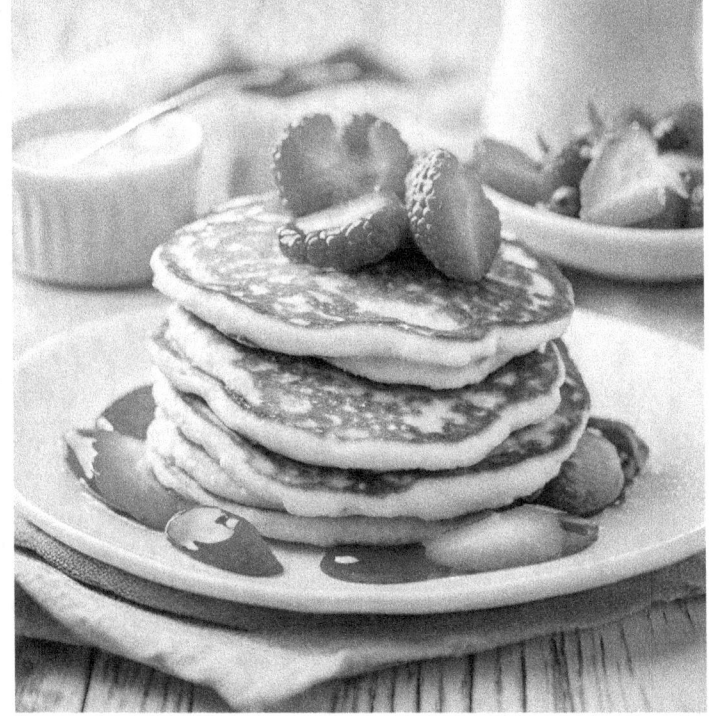

12. Whole Wheat Toast

Ingredients
- 4 slices whole wheat bread (low sodium)
- 1 tablespoon unsalted butter or olive oil (optional, for spreading)
- 1/2 avocado, sliced (optional, for topping)
- 1 medium tomato, sliced (optional, for topping)

Instructions
1. Toast the whole wheat bread slices in a toaster or on a grill until golden brown.
2. Optional: Spread a thin layer of unsalted butter or olive oil on each slice.
3. Optional: Top with avocado slices and tomato slices.
4. Serve immediately.

Nutrition Info per Serving
- Calories: 80
- Protein: 4g
- Carbohydrates: 14g
- Dietary Fiber: 3g
- Sugars: 1g
- Fat: 2g
- Saturated Fat: 0.5g
- Sodium: 80mg

Serves
4 servings

Cooking Time
5 minutes

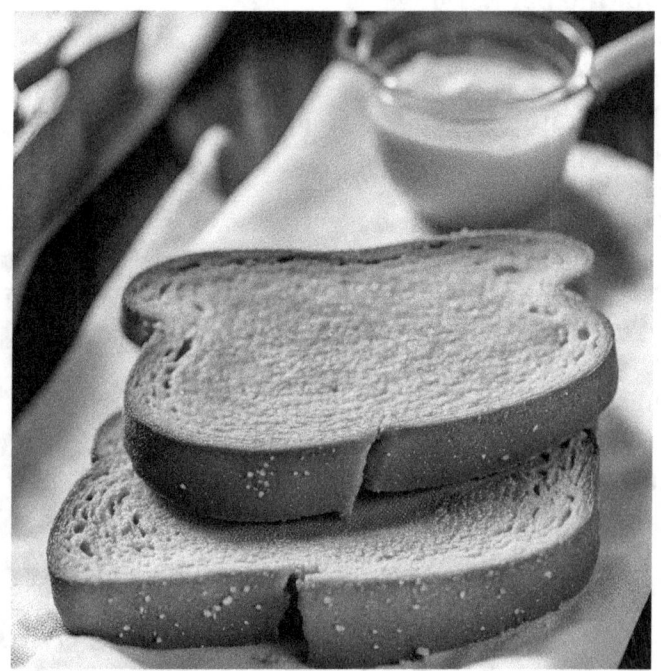

13. Almond Flour Pancakes

Ingredients
- 1 cup almond flour
- 3 large eggs
- 1/4 cup unsweetened almond milk
- 1 teaspoon baking powder (low sodium)
- 1 teaspoon vanilla extract
- 1 tablespoon honey
- 1 tablespoon olive oil (for cooking)

Instructions
1. In a large bowl, whisk together almond flour, eggs, almond milk, baking powder, vanilla extract, and honey until smooth.
2. Heat a non-stick skillet over medium heat and add a small amount of olive oil.
3. Pour 1/4 cup of batter onto the skillet for each pancake.
4. Cook for about 2-3 minutes on each side, until golden brown and cooked through.
5. Serve warm with fresh fruit or a drizzle of maple syrup.

Nutrition Info per Serving
- Calories: 180
- Protein: 7g
- Carbohydrates: 8g
- Dietary Fiber: 3g
- Sugars: 5g
- Fat: 15g
- Saturated Fat: 2g
- Sodium: 60mg

Serves
4 servings

Cooking Time
20 minutes

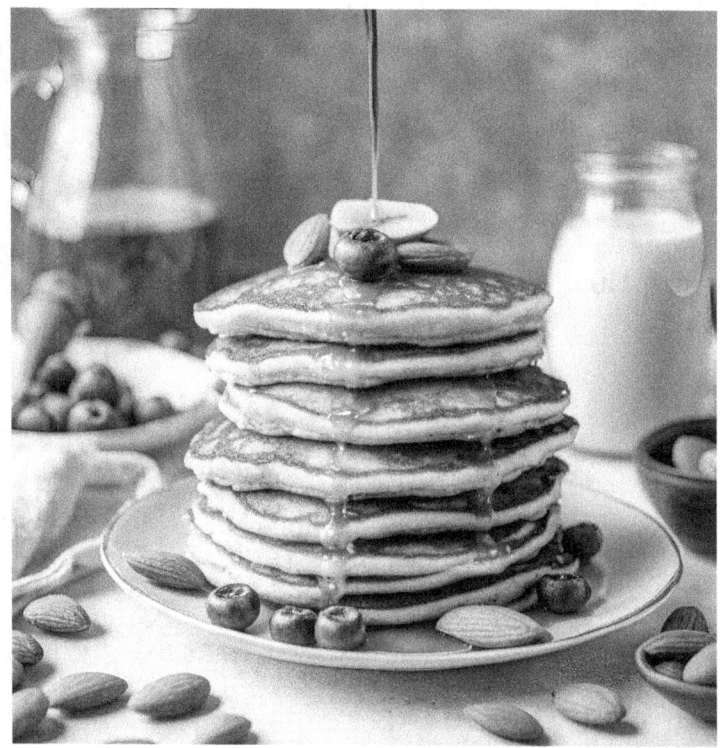

14. Buckwheat Pancakes

Ingredients
- 1 cup buckwheat flour
- 1 cup unsweetened almond milk
- 1 large egg
- 1 teaspoon baking powder (low sodium)
- 1 tablespoon honey
- 1 teaspoon vanilla extract
- 1 tablespoon olive oil (for cooking)

Instructions
1. In a large bowl, whisk together buckwheat flour, almond milk, egg, baking powder, honey, and vanilla extract until smooth.
2. Heat a non-stick skillet over medium heat and add a small amount of olive oil.
3. Pour 1/4 cup of batter onto the skillet for each pancake.
4. Cook for about 2-3 minutes on each side, until golden brown and cooked through.
5. Serve warm with fresh fruit or a drizzle of maple syrup.

Nutrition Info per Serving
- Calories: 140
- Protein: 5g
- Carbohydrates: 20g
- Dietary Fiber: 3g
- Sugars: 5g
- Fat: 5g
- Saturated Fat: 1g
- Sodium: 50mg

Serves
4 servings
Cooking Time
20 minutes

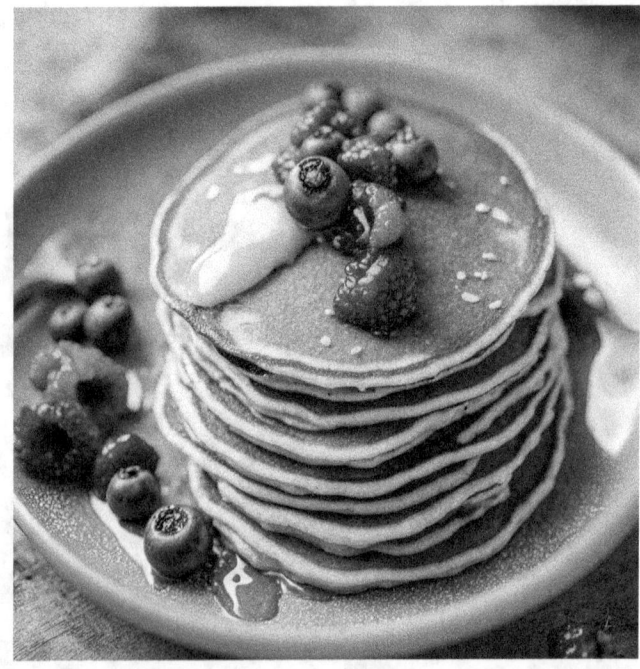

15. Oat Flour Waffles

Ingredients
- 2 cups oat flour (blend rolled oats to make flour)
- 2 large eggs
- 1 1/2 cups unsweetened almond milk
- 1 tablespoon baking powder (low sodium)
- 1 tablespoon honey
- 1 teaspoon vanilla extract
- 2 tablespoons olive oil

Instructions
1. Preheat your waffle iron according to the manufacturer's instructions.
2. In a large bowl, whisk together oat flour, eggs, almond milk, baking powder, honey, vanilla extract, and olive oil until smooth.
3. Lightly grease the waffle iron with olive oil.
4. Pour the batter into the waffle iron and cook according to the manufacturer's instructions, typically 3-5 minutes per waffle.
5. Serve warm with fresh fruit or a drizzle of maple syrup.

Nutrition Info per Serving
- Calories: 180
- Protein: 6g
- Carbohydrates: 25g
- Dietary Fiber: 4g
- Sugars: 5g
- Fat: 6g
- Saturated Fat: 1g
- Sodium: 80mg

Serves
4 servings

Cooking Time
20 minutes

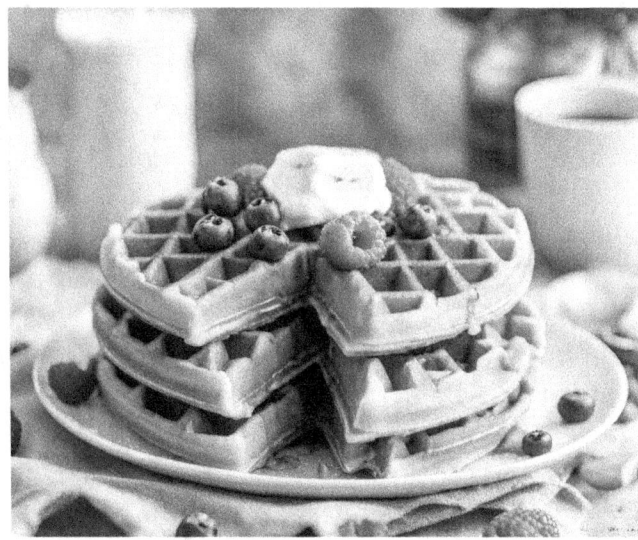

16. Frittata

Ingredients
- 6 large eggs
- 1/4 cup low-fat milk
- 1 cup spinach, chopped
- 1/2 cup cherry tomatoes, halved
- 1/4 cup red bell pepper, diced
- 1/4 cup green onions, chopped
- 1 tablespoon olive oil
- 1 teaspoon dried basil
- 1/2 teaspoon garlic powder

Instructions
1. Preheat the oven to 350°F (175°C).
2. In a large bowl, whisk together eggs and milk until well combined.
3. Stir in spinach, cherry tomatoes, red bell pepper, green onions, dried basil, and garlic powder.
4. Heat olive oil in an oven-safe skillet over medium heat.
5. Pour the egg mixture into the skillet and cook for 5-7 minutes, until the edges begin to set.
6. Transfer the skillet to the oven and bake for 15-20 minutes, until the frittata is fully set and slightly golden.
7. Let it cool slightly before slicing and serving.

Nutrition Info per Serving
- Calories: 150
- Protein: 10g
- Carbohydrates: 5g
- Dietary Fiber: 1g
- Sugars: 3g
- Fat: 10g
- Saturated Fat: 2g
- Sodium: 120mg

Serves
4 servings
Cooking Time
30 minutes

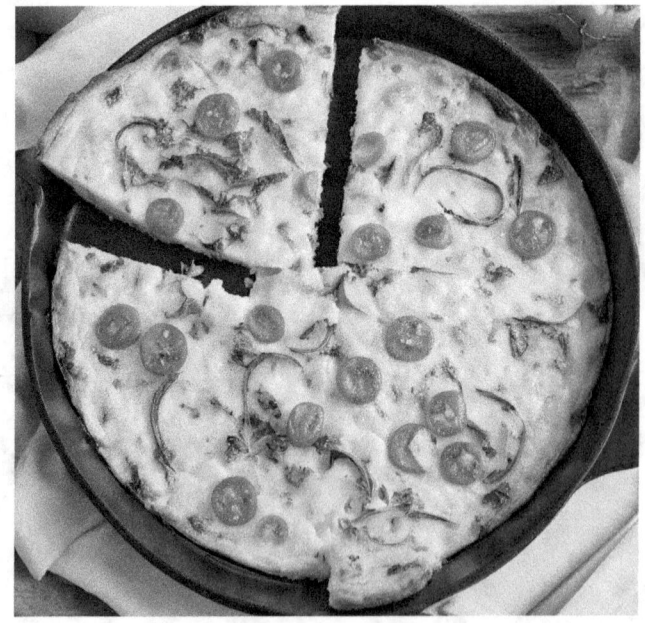

17. Egg Muffins

Ingredients
- 6 large eggs
- 1/4 cup low-fat milk
- 1/2 cup spinach, chopped
- 1/2 cup red bell pepper, diced
- 1/4 cup onion, finely chopped
- 1/4 cup mushrooms, diced
- 1 teaspoon dried oregano
- 1 tablespoon olive oil

Instructions
1. Preheat the oven to 350°F (175°C) and lightly grease a 6-cup muffin tin with olive oil.
2. In a large bowl, whisk together eggs and milk.
3. Stir in spinach, red bell pepper, onion, mushrooms, and dried oregano.
4. Pour the egg mixture evenly into the muffin cups.
5. Bake for 20-25 minutes, until the egg muffins are set and slightly golden.
6. Let them cool slightly before removing from the muffin tin and serving.

Nutrition Info per Serving
- Calories: 120
- Protein: 9g
- Carbohydrates: 4g
- Dietary Fiber: 1g
- Sugars: 2g
- Fat: 8g
- Saturated Fat: 2g
- Sodium: 90mg

Serves
6 servings

Cooking Time
30 minutes

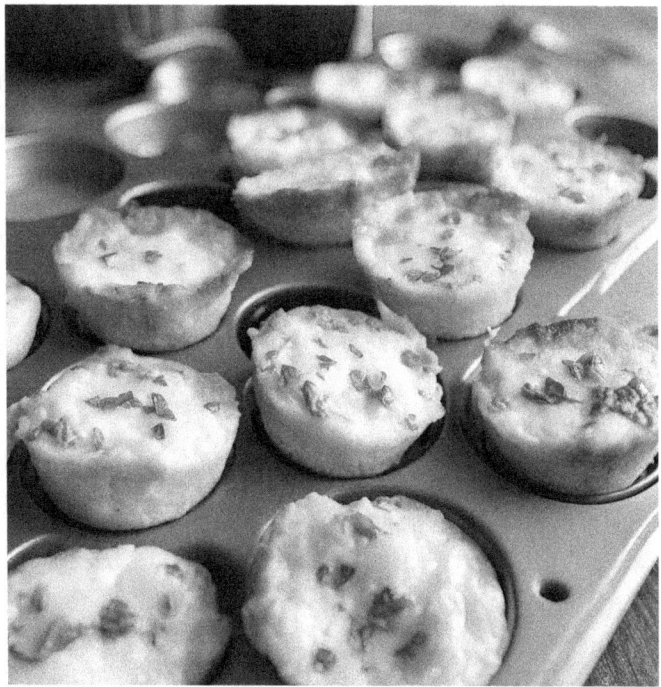

18. Barley Porridge

Ingredients
- 1 cup pearl barley
- 4 cups water
- 1/2 cup unsweetened almond milk
- 1 tablespoon honey
- 1 teaspoon ground cinnamon
- 1/4 cup chopped nuts (unsalted, optional)
- 1/4 cup fresh berries (optional)

Instructions
1. Rinse barley under cold water.
2. In a large pot, combine barley and water. Bring to a boil, then reduce heat and simmer for 40-45 minutes, until barley is tender.
3. Drain any excess water and return barley to the pot.
4. Stir in almond milk, honey, and ground cinnamon. Cook for another 5 minutes until creamy.
5. Serve warm, topped with chopped nuts and fresh berries if desired.

Nutrition Info per Serving
- Calories: 180
- Protein: 4g
- Carbohydrates: 35g
- Dietary Fiber: 6g
- Sugars: 8g
- Fat: 3g
- Saturated Fat: 0.5g
- Sodium: 10mg

Serves
4 servings
Cooking Time
50 minutes

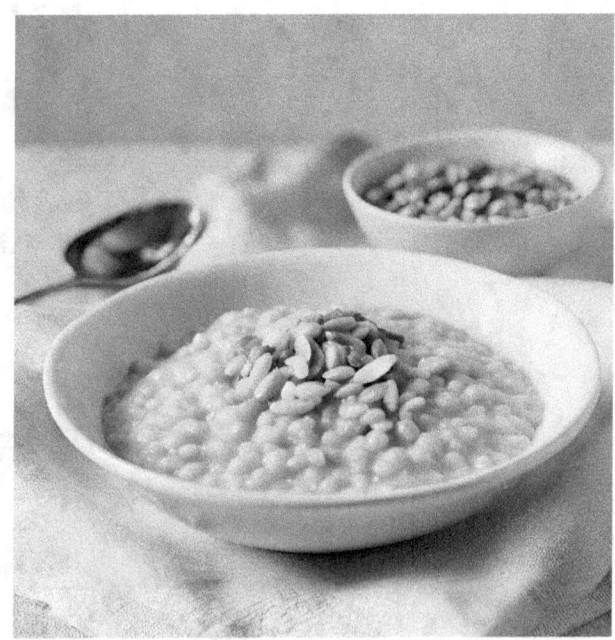

19. Buckwheat Porridge

Ingredients
- 1 cup buckwheat groats
- 3 cups water
- 1/2 cup unsweetened almond milk
- 1 tablespoon honey
- 1 teaspoon ground cinnamon
- 1/4 cup raisins
- 1/4 cup chopped nuts (unsalted, optional)

Instructions
1. Rinse buckwheat groats under cold water.
2. In a large pot, combine buckwheat and water. Bring to a boil, then reduce heat and simmer for 15-20 minutes, until buckwheat is tender.
3. Drain any excess water and return buckwheat to the pot.
4. Stir in almond milk, honey, ground cinnamon, and raisins. Cook for another 5 minutes until creamy.
5. Serve warm, topped with chopped nuts if desired.

Nutrition Info per Serving
- Calories: 190
- Protein: 5g
- Carbohydrates: 38g
- Dietary Fiber: 6g
- Sugars: 9g
- Fat: 4g
- Saturated Fat: 0.5g
- Sodium: 10mg

Serves
4 servings
Cooking Time
25 minutes

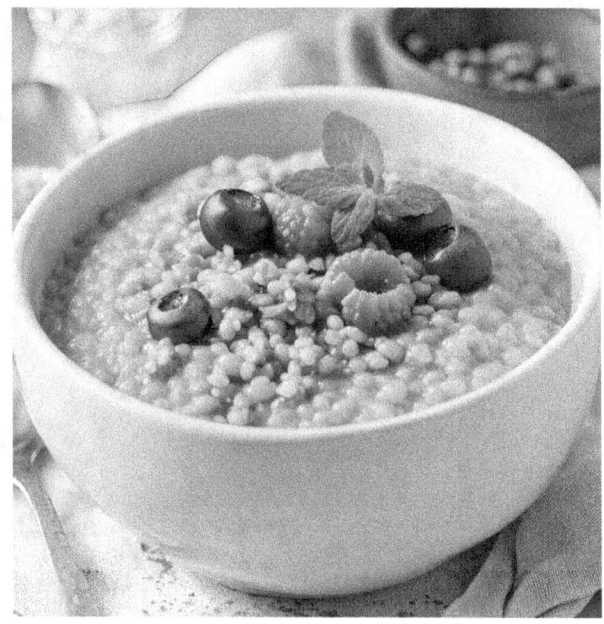

20. Quinoa Porridge

Ingredients
- 1 cup quinoa
- 2 cups water
- 1 cup unsweetened almond milk
- 1 tablespoon honey
- 1 teaspoon ground cinnamon
- 1/2 teaspoon vanilla extract
- 1/4 cup fresh berries (optional)

Instructions
1. Rinse quinoa under cold water.
2. In a medium pot, combine quinoa and water. Bring to a boil, then reduce heat and simmer for 15 minutes, until quinoa is tender and water is absorbed.
3. Stir in almond milk, honey, ground cinnamon, and vanilla extract. Cook for another 5 minutes until creamy.
4. Serve warm, topped with fresh berries if desired.

Nutrition Info per Serving
- Calories: 160
- Protein: 6g
- Carbohydrates: 28g
- Dietary Fiber: 3g
- Sugars: 8g
- Fat: 4g
- Saturated Fat: 0.5g
- Sodium: 10mg

Serves
4 servings

Cooking Time
20 minutes

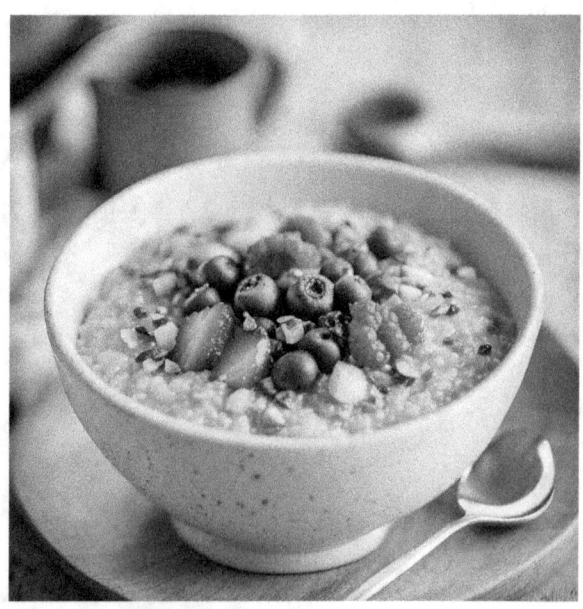

21. Avocado Smoothie

Ingredients
- 1 ripe avocado, pitted and peeled
- 1 banana
- 1 cup unsweetened almond milk
- 1 tablespoon honey
- 1 teaspoon vanilla extract
- 1 cup ice cubes

Instructions
1. In a blender, combine avocado, banana, almond milk, honey, vanilla extract, and ice cubes.
2. Blend until smooth and creamy.
3. Pour into glasses and serve immediately.

Nutrition Info per Serving
Calories: 220 Protein: 2g Carbohydrates: 32g Dietary Fiber: 6g Sugars: 18g
- Fat: 10g Saturated Fat: 1.5g Sodium: 10mg

Serves
2 servings

Cooking Time
5 minutes

22. Berry Banana Smoothie

Ingredients
- 1 banana
- 1/2 cup strawberries
- 1/2 cup blueberries
- 1/2 cup raspberries
- 1 cup unsweetened almond milk
- 1 tablespoon honey
- 1 cup ice cubes

Instructions
1. In a blender, combine banana, strawberries, blueberries, raspberries, almond milk, honey, and ice cubes.
2. Blend until smooth and creamy.
3. Pour into glasses and serve immediately.

Nutrition Info per Serving
- Calories: 160 Protein: 2g Carbohydrates: 35g Dietary Fiber: 7g
- Sugars: 22g Fat: 2g Saturated Fat: 0.5g Sodium: 10mg

Serves
2 servings

Cooking Time
5 minutes

23. Pineapple Coconut Smoothie

Ingredients
- 1 cup pineapple chunks
- 1/2 banana
- 1 cup coconut water
- 1/2 cup unsweetened coconut milk
- 1 tablespoon honey
- 1 cup ice cubes

Instructions
1. In a blender, combine pineapple chunks, banana, coconut water, coconut milk, honey, and ice cubes.
2. Blend until smooth and creamy.
3. Pour into glasses and serve immediately.

Nutrition Info per Serving
- Calories: 150
- Protein: 1g
- Carbohydrates: 35g
- Dietary Fiber: 3g
- Sugars: 28g
- Fat: 2g
- Saturated Fat: 1.5g
- Sodium: 20mg

Serves
2 servings

Cooking Time
5 minutes

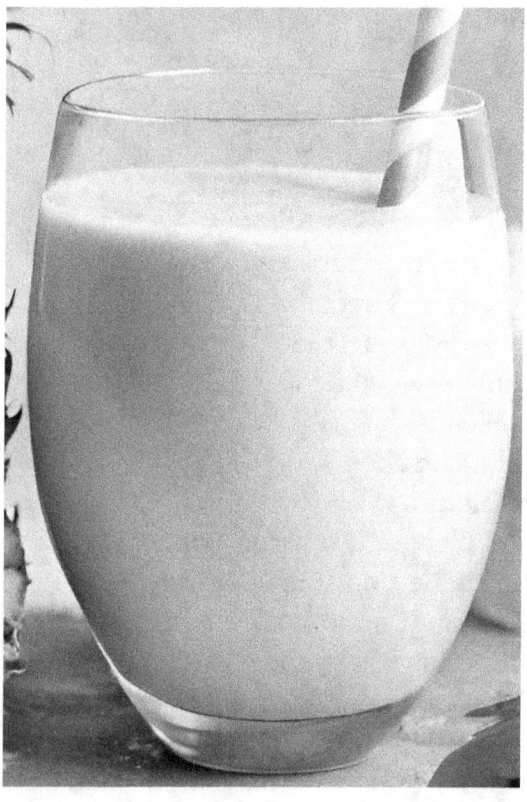

Fish & Seafood Recipes

1. Lemon Herb Baked Cod

Ingredients
- 4 cod fillets (about 6 ounces each)
- 2 tablespoons olive oil
- 2 tablespoons fresh lemon juice
- 2 teaspoons lemon zest
- 1 teaspoon dried thyme
- 1 teaspoon dried parsley
- 2 cloves garlic, minced
- Fresh lemon slices for garnish

Instructions
1. Preheat the oven to 375°F (190°C).
2. In a small bowl, mix together olive oil, lemon juice, lemon zest, dried thyme, dried parsley, and minced garlic.
3. Place the cod fillets in a baking dish and brush the lemon herb mixture evenly over the fillets.
4. Bake in the preheated oven for 15-20 minutes, or until the fish is opaque and flakes easily with a fork.
5. Garnish with fresh lemon slices and serve immediately.

Nutrition Info per Serving
- Calories: 200
- Protein: 35g
- Carbohydrates: 1g
- Dietary Fiber: 0g
- Sugars: 0g
- Fat: 6g
- Saturated Fat: 1g
- Sodium: 75mg

Serves
4 servings

Cooking Time
25 minutes

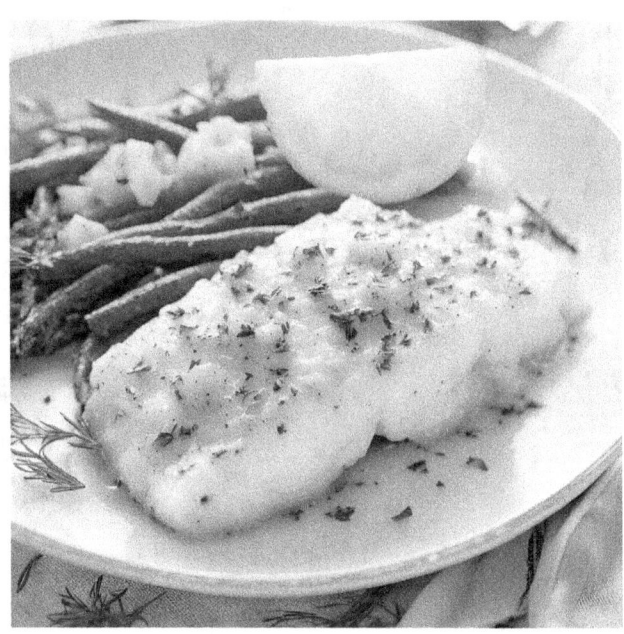

2. Roasted Salmon with Dill

Ingredients
- 4 salmon fillets (about 6 ounces each)
- 2 tablespoons olive oil
- 2 tablespoons fresh lemon juice
- 2 teaspoons dried dill
- 2 cloves garlic, minced
- Fresh dill sprigs for garnish

Instructions
1. Preheat the oven to 400°F (200°C).
2. In a small bowl, mix together olive oil, lemon juice, dried dill, and minced garlic.
3. Place the salmon fillets on a baking sheet lined with parchment paper and brush the olive oil mixture evenly over the fillets.
4. Bake in the preheated oven for 12-15 minutes, or until the salmon is opaque and flakes easily with a fork.
5. Garnish with fresh dill sprigs and serve immediately.

Nutrition Info per Serving
- Calories: 290
- Protein: 34g
- Carbohydrates: 1g
- Dietary Fiber: 0g
- Sugars: 0g
- Fat: 17g
- Saturated Fat: 3g
- Sodium: 70mg

Serves
4 servings

Cooking Time
20 minutes

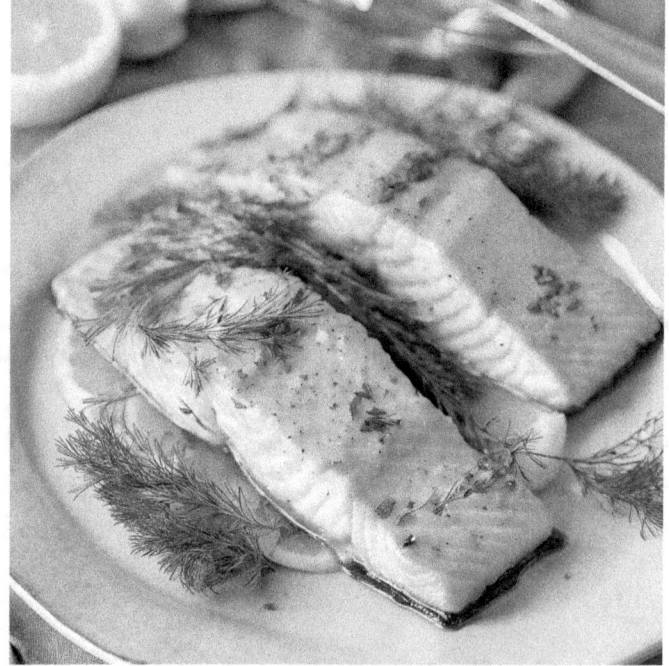

3. Paprika Tilapia

Ingredients
- 4 tilapia fillets (about 6 ounces each)
- 2 tablespoons olive oil
- 1 teaspoon paprika
- 1 teaspoon garlic powder
- 1 teaspoon onion powder
- 1 teaspoon dried oregano
- 1 tablespoon fresh lemon juice
- Fresh parsley for garnish

Instructions
1. Preheat the oven to 375°F (190°C).
2. In a small bowl, mix together olive oil, paprika, garlic powder, onion powder, dried oregano, and lemon juice.
3. Place the tilapia fillets in a baking dish and brush the paprika mixture evenly over the fillets.
4. Bake in the preheated oven for 15-20 minutes, or until the fish is opaque and flakes easily with a fork.
5. Garnish with fresh parsley and serve immediately.

Nutrition Info per Serving
- Calories: 190
- Protein: 35g
- Carbohydrates: 1g
- Dietary Fiber: 0g
- Sugars: 0g
- Fat: 5g
- Saturated Fat: 1g
- Sodium: 60mg

Serves
4 servings

Cooking Time
25 minutes

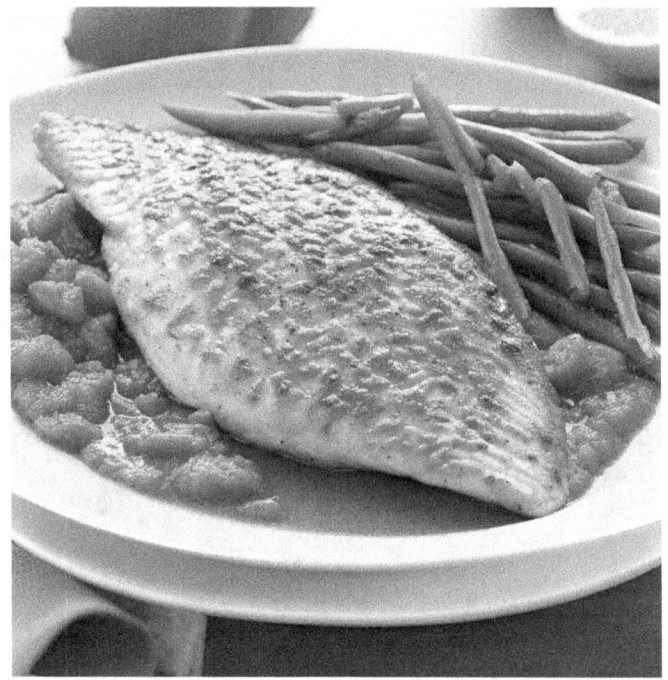

4. Baked Haddock with Tomatoes

Ingredients
- 4 haddock fillets (about 6 ounces each)
- 2 tablespoons olive oil
- 2 cups cherry tomatoes, halved
- 2 cloves garlic, minced
- 1 teaspoon dried basil
- 1 teaspoon dried oregano
- 1 tablespoon fresh lemon juice
- Fresh basil leaves for garnish

Instructions
1. Preheat the oven to 375°F (190°C).
2. In a small bowl, mix together olive oil, garlic, dried basil, dried oregano, and lemon juice.
3. Place the haddock fillets in a baking dish and arrange the cherry tomatoes around them.
4. Brush the olive oil mixture evenly over the fillets and tomatoes.
5. Bake in the preheated oven for 20-25 minutes, or until the fish is opaque and flakes easily with a fork and the tomatoes are soft.
6. Garnish with fresh basil leaves and serve immediately.

Nutrition Info per Serving
- Calories: 210
- Protein: 36g
- Carbohydrates: 3g
- Dietary Fiber: 1g
- Sugars: 2g
- Fat: 6g
- Saturated Fat: 1g
- Sodium: 75mg

Serves
4 servings

Cooking Time
30 minutes

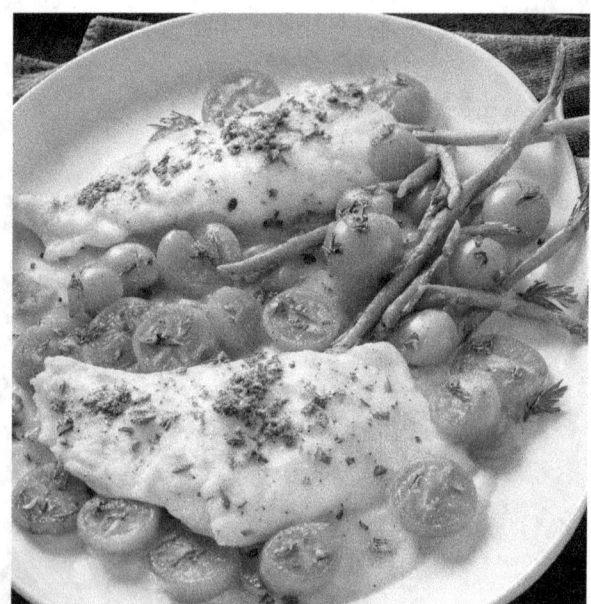

5. Mustard Roasted Trout

Ingredients
- 4 trout fillets (about 6 ounces each)
- 2 tablespoons Dijon mustard (low sodium)
- 1 tablespoon honey
- 2 tablespoons olive oil
- 2 cloves garlic, minced
- 1 teaspoon dried thyme
- 1 teaspoon paprika

Instructions
1. Preheat the oven to 375°F (190°C).
2. In a small bowl, mix together Dijon mustard, honey, olive oil, garlic, thyme, and paprika.
3. Place the trout fillets in a baking dish and brush the mustard mixture evenly over the fillets.
4. Bake in the preheated oven for 15-20 minutes, or until the fish is opaque and flakes easily with a fork.
5. Serve immediately.

Nutrition Info per Serving
- Calories: 250
- Protein: 36g
- Carbohydrates: 5g
- Dietary Fiber: 1g
- Sugars: 3g
- Fat: 10g
- Saturated Fat: 2g
- Sodium: 70mg

Serves
4 servings

Cooking Time
25 minutes

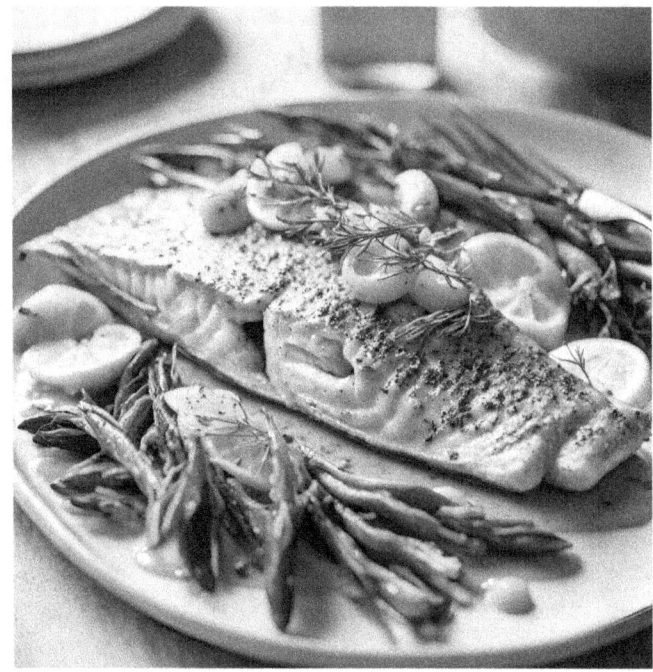

6. Orange Glazed Halibut

Ingredients
- 4 halibut fillets (about 6 ounces each)
- 1/4 cup fresh orange juice
- 1 tablespoon orange zest
- 2 tablespoons honey
- 1 tablespoon olive oil
- 2 cloves garlic, minced
- 1 teaspoon dried rosemary

Instructions
1. Preheat the oven to 400°F (200°C).
2. In a small bowl, mix together orange juice, orange zest, honey, olive oil, garlic, and rosemary.
3. Place the halibut fillets in a baking dish and pour the orange mixture over the fillets.
4. Bake in the preheated oven for 12-15 minutes, or until the fish is opaque and flakes easily with a fork.
5. Serve immediately.

Nutrition Info per Serving
- Calories: 270
- Protein: 34g
- Carbohydrates: 10g
- Dietary Fiber: 1g
- Sugars: 9g
- Fat: 10g
- Saturated Fat: 2g
- Sodium: 60mg

Serves
4 servings

Cooking Time
20 minutes

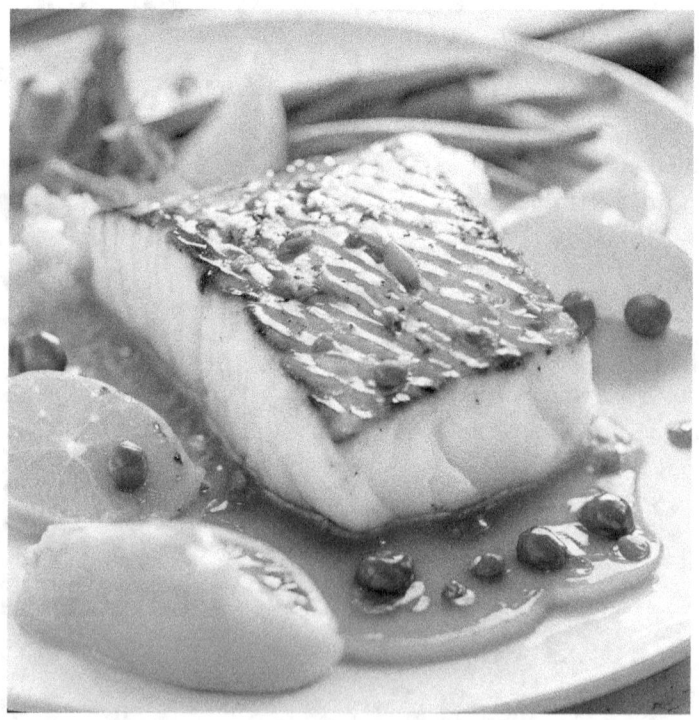

7. Lemon Pepper Catfish

Ingredients
- 4 catfish fillets (about 6 ounces each)
- 2 tablespoons olive oil
- 1 tablespoon lemon juice
- 1 tablespoon lemon zest
- 1 teaspoon freshly ground black pepper
- 1 teaspoon garlic powder
- 1 teaspoon dried parsley

Instructions
1. Preheat the oven to 375°F (190°C).
2. In a small bowl, mix together olive oil, lemon juice, lemon zest, black pepper, garlic powder, and dried parsley.
3. Place the catfish fillets in a baking dish and brush the lemon pepper mixture evenly over the fillets.
4. Bake in the preheated oven for 15-20 minutes, or until the fish is opaque and flakes easily with a fork.
5. Serve immediately.

Nutrition Info per Serving
- Calories: 220
- Protein: 32g
- Carbohydrates: 2g
- Dietary Fiber: 1g
- Sugars: 0g
- Fat: 9g
- Saturated Fat: 1.5g
- Sodium: 60mg

Serves
4 servings

Cooking Time
25 minutes

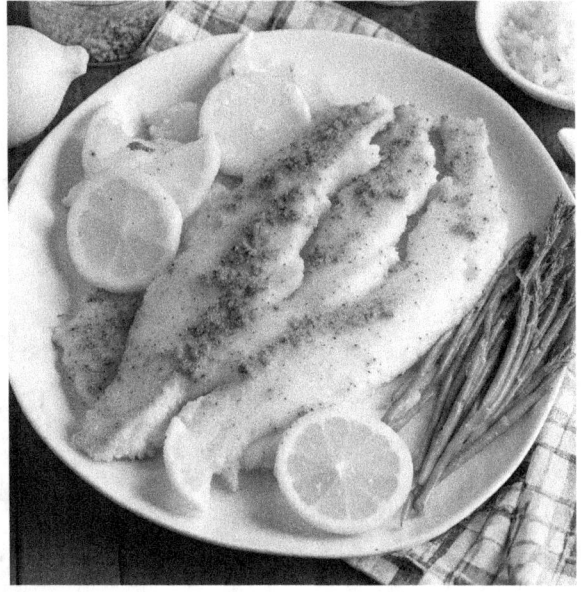

8. Herbed Sea Bass

Ingredients
- 4 sea bass fillets (about 6 ounces each)
- 2 tablespoons olive oil
- 2 cloves garlic, minced
- 1 tablespoon fresh lemon juice
- 1 teaspoon dried thyme
- 1 teaspoon dried oregano
- 1 teaspoon dried basil

Instructions
1. Preheat the oven to 375°F (190°C).
2. In a small bowl, mix together olive oil, garlic, lemon juice, thyme, oregano, and basil.
3. Place the sea bass fillets in a baking dish and brush the herb mixture evenly over the fillets.
4. Bake in the preheated oven for 15-20 minutes, or until the fish is opaque and flakes easily with a fork.
5. Serve immediately.

Nutrition Info per Serving
- Calories: 230
- Protein: 35g
- Carbohydrates: 2g
- Dietary Fiber: 1g
- Sugars: 0g
- Fat: 9g
- Saturated Fat: 1.5g
- Sodium: 65mg

Serves
4 servings

Cooking Time
25 minutes

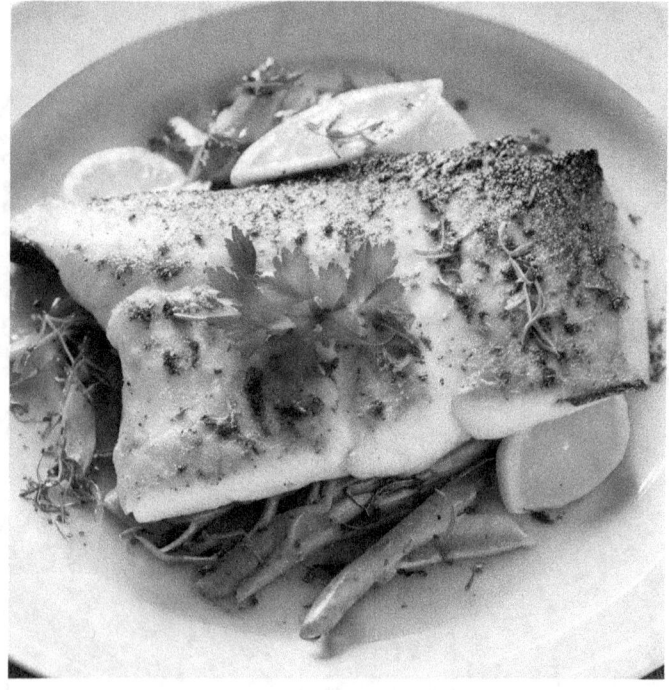

9. Baked Scallops with Herbs

Ingredients
- 1 pound sea scallops
- 2 tablespoons olive oil
- 2 cloves garlic, minced
- 1 tablespoon fresh lemon juice
- 1 teaspoon dried parsley
- 1 teaspoon dried thyme
- 1 teaspoon paprika

Instructions
1. Preheat the oven to 400°F (200°C).
2. In a small bowl, mix together olive oil, garlic, lemon juice, parsley, thyme, and paprika.
3. Place the scallops in a baking dish and pour the herb mixture over them, tossing gently to coat.
4. Bake in the preheated oven for 10-12 minutes, or until the scallops are opaque and slightly firm.
5. Serve immediately.

Nutrition Info per Serving
- Calories: 200
- Protein: 24g
- Carbohydrates: 3g
- Dietary Fiber: 1g
- Sugars: 0g
- Fat: 10g
- Saturated Fat: 1.5g
- Sodium: 80mg

Serves
4 servings
Cooking Time
15 minutes

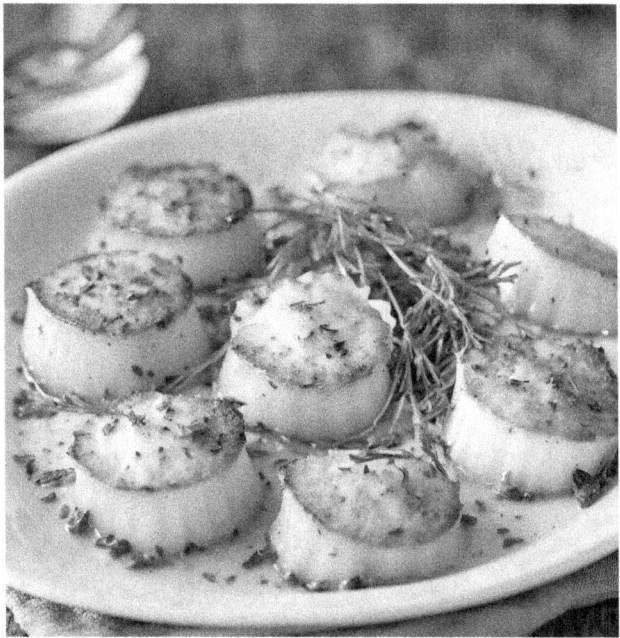

10. Grilled Mackerel with Lime

Ingredients
- 4 mackerel fillets (about 6 ounces each)
- 2 tablespoons olive oil
- 1 tablespoon fresh lime juice
- 1 teaspoon lime zest
- 2 cloves garlic, minced
- 1 teaspoon ground cumin
- Fresh cilantro for garnish

Instructions
1. Preheat the grill to medium-high heat.
2. In a small bowl, mix together olive oil, lime juice, lime zest, garlic, and ground cumin.
3. Brush the mackerel fillets with the lime mixture.
4. Grill the mackerel fillets for 5-7 minutes on each side, or until the fish is opaque and flakes easily with a fork.
5. Garnish with fresh cilantro and serve immediately.

Nutrition Info per Serving
- Calories: 250
- Protein: 34g
- Carbohydrates: 1g
- Dietary Fiber: 0g
- Sugars: 0g
- Fat: 12g
- Saturated Fat: 3g
- Sodium: 70mg

Serves
4 servings

Cooking Time
15 minutes

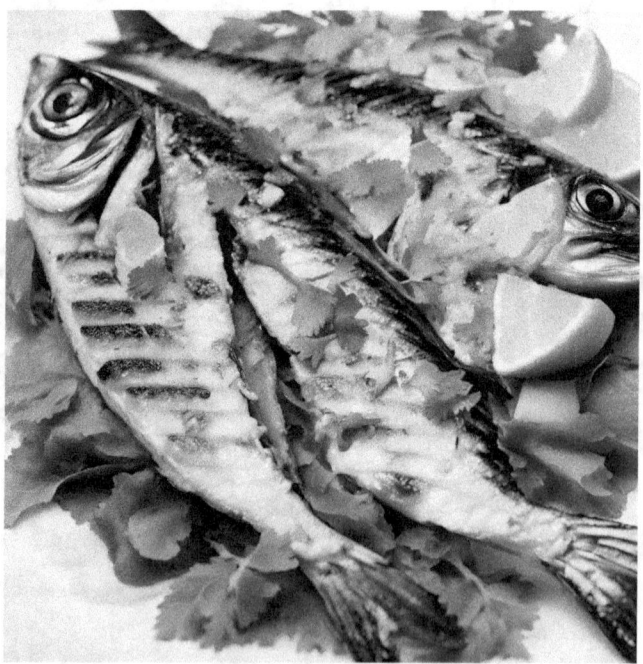

11. Grilled Sardines with Lemon

Ingredients
- 12 fresh sardines, cleaned and scaled
- 3 tablespoons olive oil
- 2 tablespoons fresh lemon juice
- 2 cloves garlic, minced
- 1 teaspoon dried oregano
- Lemon wedges for serving
- Fresh parsley for garnish

Instructions
1. Preheat the grill to medium-high heat.
2. In a small bowl, mix together olive oil, lemon juice, garlic, and oregano.
3. Brush the sardines with the olive oil mixture.
4. Grill the sardines for 3-4 minutes on each side, or until they are cooked through and have nice grill marks.
5. Garnish with fresh parsley and serve with lemon wedges.

Nutrition Info per Serving
- Calories: 220
- Protein: 26g
- Carbohydrates: 1g
- Dietary Fiber: 0g
- Sugars: 0g
- Fat: 12g
- Saturated Fat: 2g
- Sodium: 80mg

Serves
4 servings

Cooking Time
15 minutes

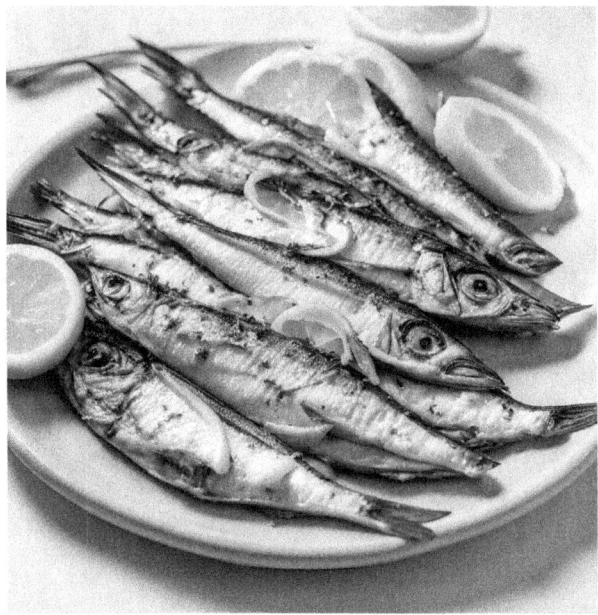

12. Grilled Tuna with Basil Pesto

Ingredients
- 4 tuna steaks (about 6 ounces each)
- 3 tablespoons olive oil
- 1 cup fresh basil leaves
- 2 cloves garlic
- 1/4 cup unsalted pine nuts
- 1/4 cup grated Parmesan cheese (low sodium or homemade)
- 1 tablespoon fresh lemon juice

Instructions
1. Preheat the grill to medium-high heat.
2. Brush the tuna steaks with 1 tablespoon of olive oil.
3. Grill the tuna steaks for 3-4 minutes on each side, or until desired doneness.
4. While the tuna is grilling, make the basil pesto. In a food processor, combine basil leaves, garlic, pine nuts, Parmesan cheese, and lemon juice. Blend until smooth, slowly adding the remaining olive oil until well combined.
5. Serve the grilled tuna with a dollop of basil pesto on top.

Nutrition Info per Serving
- Calories: 350
- Protein: 34g
- Carbohydrates: 2g
- Dietary Fiber: 1g
- Sugars: 0g
- Fat: 24g
- Saturated Fat: 4g
- Sodium: 110mg

Serves
4 servings
Cooking Time
15 minutes

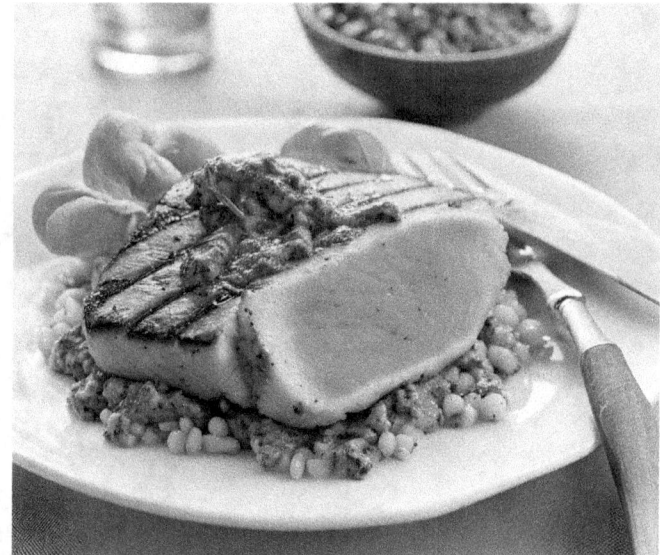

13. Chili Lime Shrimp Skewers

Ingredients
- 1 pound large shrimp, peeled and deveined
- 3 tablespoons olive oil
- 2 tablespoons fresh lime juice
- 1 teaspoon lime zest
- 1 teaspoon chili powder
- 2 cloves garlic, minced
- Fresh cilantro for garnish

Instructions
1. Preheat the grill to medium-high heat.
2. In a large bowl, combine olive oil, lime juice, lime zest, chili powder, and garlic. Add the shrimp and toss to coat.
3. Thread the shrimp onto skewers.
4. Grill the shrimp skewers for 2-3 minutes on each side, or until the shrimp are opaque and cooked through.
5. Garnish with fresh cilantro and serve immediately.

Nutrition Info per Serving
- Calories: 180
- Protein: 23g
- Carbohydrates: 2g
- Dietary Fiber: 1g
- Sugars: 0g
- Fat: 9g
- Saturated Fat: 1.5g
- Sodium: 150mg

Serves
4 servings
Cooking Time
10 minutes

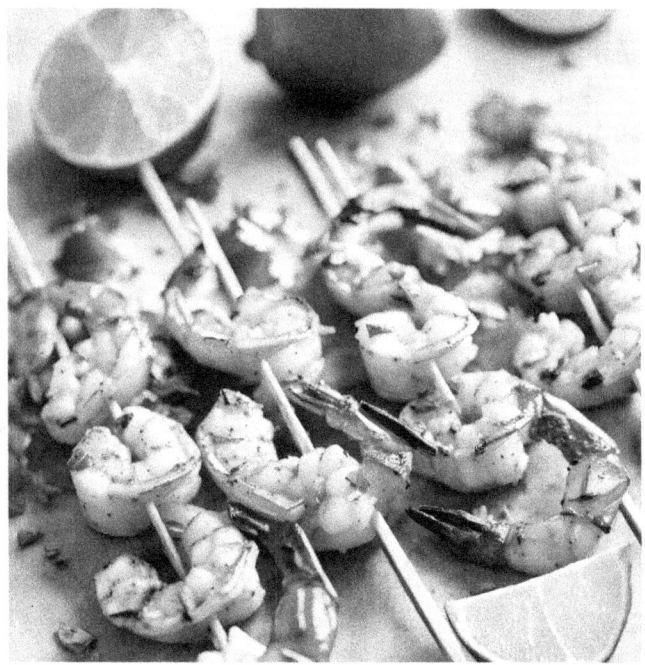

14. Grilled Swordfish with Salsa Verde

Ingredients
- 4 swordfish steaks (about 6 ounces each)
- 3 tablespoons olive oil
- 1 tablespoon fresh lemon juice
- 1 cup fresh parsley, chopped
- 1/4 cup fresh mint leaves, chopped
- 2 cloves garlic, minced
- 2 tablespoons capers, rinsed and chopped
- 2 tablespoons red wine vinegar
- Lemon wedges for serving

Instructions
1. Preheat the grill to medium-high heat.
2. Brush the swordfish steaks with 1 tablespoon of olive oil and lemon juice.
3. Grill the swordfish steaks for 4-5 minutes on each side, or until they are opaque and cooked through.
4. While the fish is grilling, prepare the salsa verde. In a bowl, combine parsley, mint, garlic, capers, remaining olive oil, and red wine vinegar. Mix well.
5. Serve the grilled swordfish topped with salsa verde and lemon wedges on the side.

Nutrition Info per Serving
- Calories: 280
- Protein: 36g
- Carbohydrates: 3g
- Dietary Fiber: 1g
- Sugars: 0g
- Fat: 14g
- Saturated Fat: 2g
- Sodium: 80mg

Serves
4 servings

Cooking Time
15 minutes

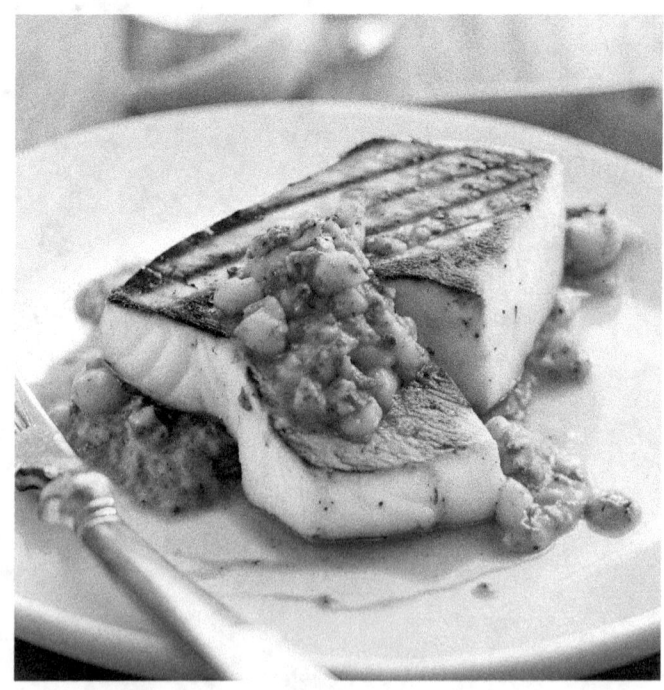

15. Grilled Clams with Garlic

Ingredients
- 2 pounds fresh clams, scrubbed clean
- 3 tablespoons olive oil
- 4 cloves garlic, minced
- 1/4 cup fresh parsley, chopped
- Juice of 1 lemon
- Lemon wedges for serving

Instructions
1. Preheat the grill to medium-high heat.
2. In a small bowl, mix together olive oil, garlic, parsley, and lemon juice.
3. Place the clams on a large piece of aluminum foil, forming a packet. Pour the garlic mixture over the clams.
4. Close the foil packet tightly and place it on the grill.
5. Grill for 10-12 minutes, or until the clams open. Discard any clams that do not open.
6. Serve immediately with lemon wedges.

Nutrition Info per Serving
- Calories: 200
- Protein: 26g
- Carbohydrates: 4g
- Dietary Fiber: 0g
- Sugars: 0g
- Fat: 8g
- Saturated Fat: 1g
- Sodium: 90mg

Serves
4 servings

Cooking Time
15 minutes

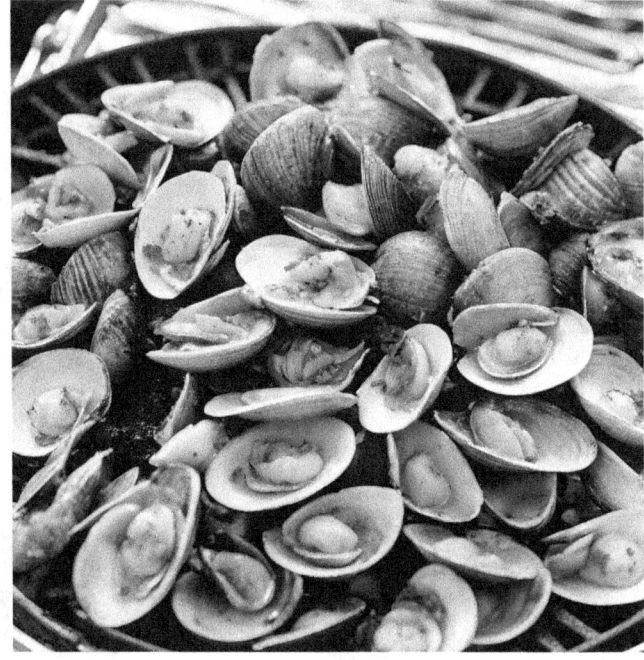

16. Broiled Tilapia with Thyme

Ingredients
- 4 tilapia fillets (about 6 ounces each)
- 3 tablespoons olive oil
- 1 tablespoon fresh lemon juice
- 2 cloves garlic, minced
- 1 teaspoon dried thyme
- Fresh thyme sprigs for garnish
- Lemon wedges for serving

Instructions
1. Preheat the broiler.
2. In a small bowl, mix together olive oil, lemon juice, garlic, and dried thyme.
3. Place the tilapia fillets on a broiler pan and brush with the olive oil mixture.
4. Broil for 5-6 minutes, or until the fish is opaque and flakes easily with a fork.
5. Garnish with fresh thyme sprigs and serve with lemon wedges.

Nutrition Info per Serving
- Calories: 210
- Protein: 34g
- Carbohydrates: 2g
- Dietary Fiber: 0g
- Sugars: 0g
- Fat: 8g
- Saturated Fat: 1.5g
- Sodium: 70mg

Serves
4 servings
Cooking Time
10 minutes

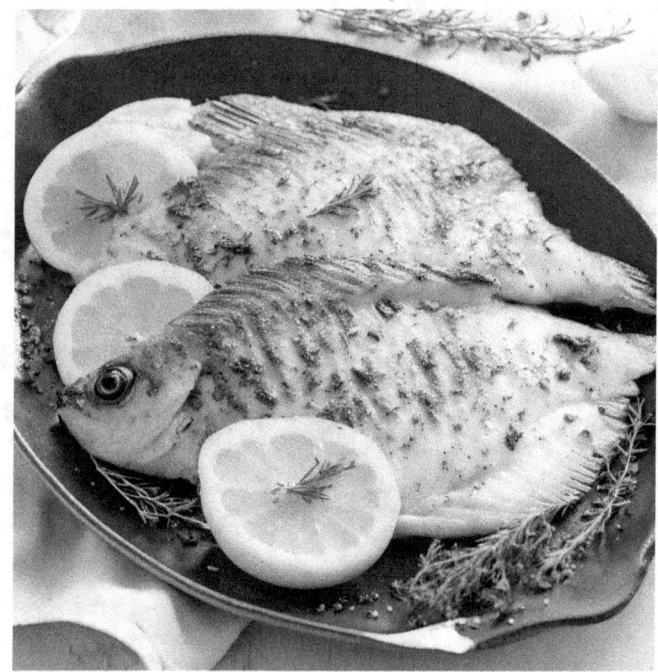

17. Tom Yum Goong

Ingredients
- 1 pound large shrimp, peeled and deveined
- 4 cups low-sodium chicken broth
- 2 stalks lemongrass, cut into 2-inch pieces and smashed
- 3 kaffir lime leaves, torn into pieces
- 1 inch piece of galangal, sliced
- 2 cloves garlic, minced
- 2-3 Thai chilies, sliced
- 1 cup mushrooms, sliced
- 1 medium tomato, cut into wedges
- 2 tablespoons fish sauce (low sodium, or homemade)
- 1 tablespoon lime juice
- 1 tablespoon low-sodium soy sauce
- Fresh cilantro for garnish

Instructions
1. In a large pot, bring the chicken broth to a boil.
2. Add lemongrass, kaffir lime leaves, galangal, garlic, and Thai chilies. Simmer for 5-10 minutes to infuse the flavors.
3. Add the mushrooms and tomato, and cook for another 5 minutes.
4. Add the shrimp and cook until they turn pink and are cooked through, about 3-4 minutes.
5. Stir in the fish sauce, lime juice, and soy sauce.
6. Remove from heat and garnish with fresh cilantro before serving.

Nutrition Info per Serving
- Calories: 150
- Protein: 22g
- Carbohydrates: 4g
- Dietary Fiber: 1g
- Sugars: 2g
- Fat: 4g
- Saturated Fat: 1g
- Sodium: 150mg

Serves
4 servings
Cooking Time
20 minutes

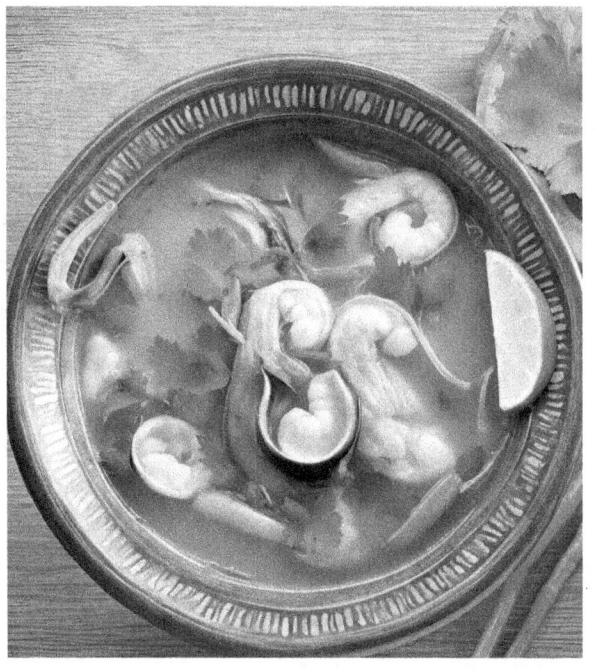

18. Pan-Seared Scallops with Lemon

Ingredients
- 1 pound large sea scallops
- 2 tablespoons olive oil
- 2 tablespoons fresh lemon juice
- 1 teaspoon lemon zest
- 2 cloves garlic, minced
- 1 tablespoon fresh parsley, chopped
- Lemon wedges for serving

Instructions
1. Pat the scallops dry with paper towels.
2. Heat olive oil in a large skillet over medium-high heat.
3. Add scallops to the skillet and cook for 2-3 minutes on each side until they are golden brown and opaque.
4. Add garlic and cook for an additional minute.
5. Remove the skillet from heat and stir in lemon juice and lemon zest.
6. Sprinkle with fresh parsley.
7. Serve immediately with lemon wedges.

Nutrition Info per Serving
- Calories: 220
- Protein: 26g
- Carbohydrates: 3g
- Dietary Fiber: 1g
- Sugars: 0g
- Fat: 11g
- Saturated Fat: 2g
- Sodium: 140mg

Serves
4 servings

Cooking Time
10 minutes

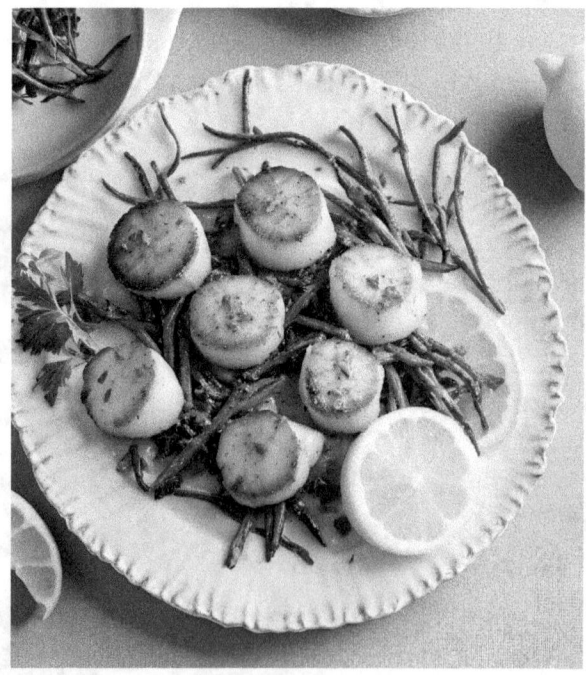

19. Lemon Sole Meuniere

Ingredients
- 4 sole fillets (about 6 ounces each)
- 1/4 cup whole wheat flour
- 3 tablespoons unsalted butter
- 2 tablespoons fresh lemon juice
- 1 teaspoon lemon zest
- 1 tablespoon fresh parsley, chopped
- 2 tablespoons olive oil
- Lemon wedges for serving

Instructions
1. Dredge the sole fillets in flour, shaking off any excess.
2. Heat 2 tablespoons of olive oil and 1 tablespoon of butter in a large skillet over medium heat.
3. Add the sole fillets to the skillet and cook for 2-3 minutes on each side until golden brown.
4. Remove the fillets from the skillet and keep warm.
5. In the same skillet, add the remaining butter and melt over medium heat.
6. Stir in lemon juice and lemon zest.
7. Pour the sauce over the cooked sole fillets.
8. Garnish with fresh parsley and serve immediately with lemon wedges.

Nutrition Info per Serving
- Calories: 280
- Protein: 28g
- Carbohydrates: 5g
- Dietary Fiber: 1g
- Sugars: 0g
- Fat: 17g
- Saturated Fat: 7g
- Sodium: 120mg

Serves
4 servings

Cooking Time
15 minutes

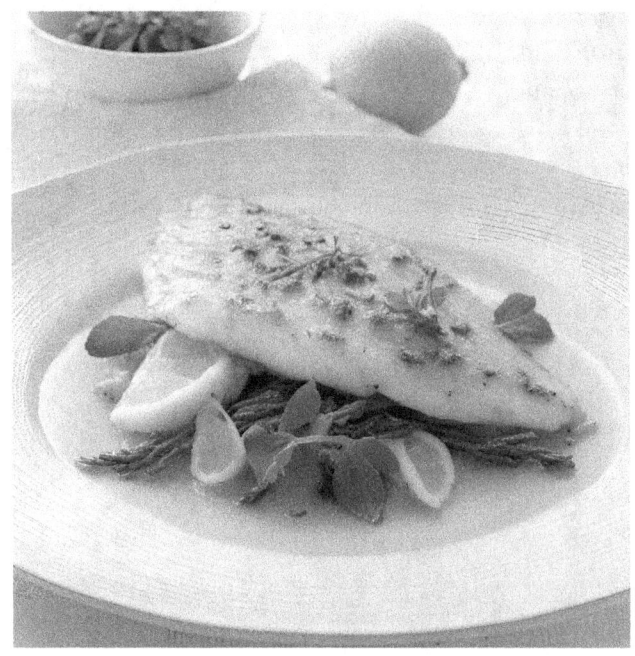

20. Peppered Mackerel

Ingredients
- 4 mackerel fillets (about 6 ounces each)
- 2 tablespoons olive oil
- 2 cloves garlic, minced
- 1 teaspoon freshly ground black pepper
- 1 tablespoon fresh lemon juice
- Fresh parsley for garnish

Instructions
1. Preheat the oven to 375°F (190°C).
2. In a small bowl, mix together olive oil, garlic, black pepper, and lemon juice.
3. Place the mackerel fillets in a baking dish and brush the olive oil mixture evenly over the fillets.
4. Bake in the preheated oven for 15-20 minutes, or until the fish is opaque and flakes easily with a fork.
5. Garnish with fresh parsley and serve immediately.

Nutrition Info per Serving
- Calories: 260
- Protein: 28g
- Carbohydrates: 1g
- Dietary Fiber: 0g
- Sugars: 0g
- Fat: 16g
- Saturated Fat: 3g
- Sodium: 75mg

Serves
4 servings
Cooking Time
20 minute

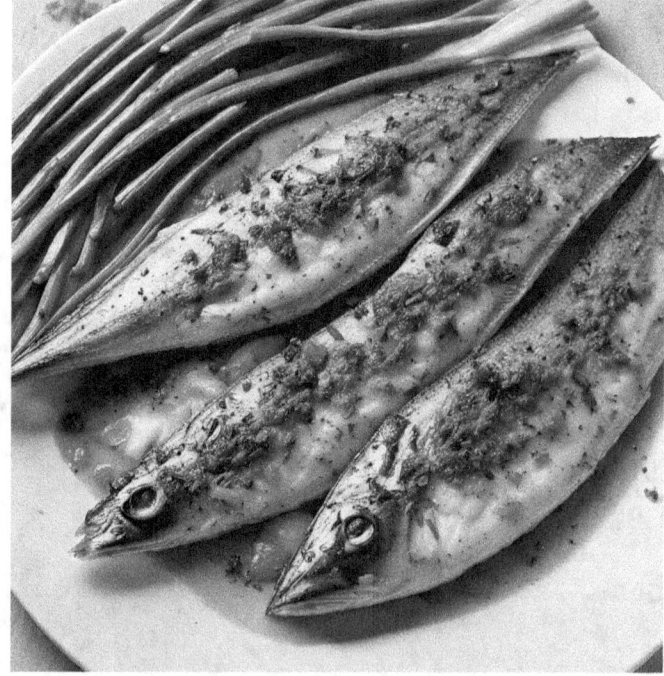

21. Sautéed Shrimp with Ginger and Honey

Ingredients
- 1 pound large shrimp, peeled and deveined
- 2 tablespoons olive oil
- 2 tablespoons honey
- 1 tablespoon fresh ginger, grated
- 2 cloves garlic, minced
- 1 tablespoon fresh lemon juice
- Fresh cilantro for garnish

Instructions
1. In a large skillet, heat olive oil over medium-high heat.
2. Add garlic and ginger, and sauté for about 1 minute until fragrant.
3. Add shrimp to the skillet and cook for 2-3 minutes on each side until they turn pink and are cooked through.
4. Drizzle honey and lemon juice over the shrimp and toss to coat.
5. Garnish with fresh cilantro and serve immediately.

Nutrition Info per Serving
- Calories: 220
- Protein: 24g
- Carbohydrates: 12g
- Dietary Fiber: 0g
- Sugars: 11g
- Fat: 9g
- Saturated Fat: 1.5g
- Sodium: 140mg

Serves
4 servings
Cooking Time
10 minutes

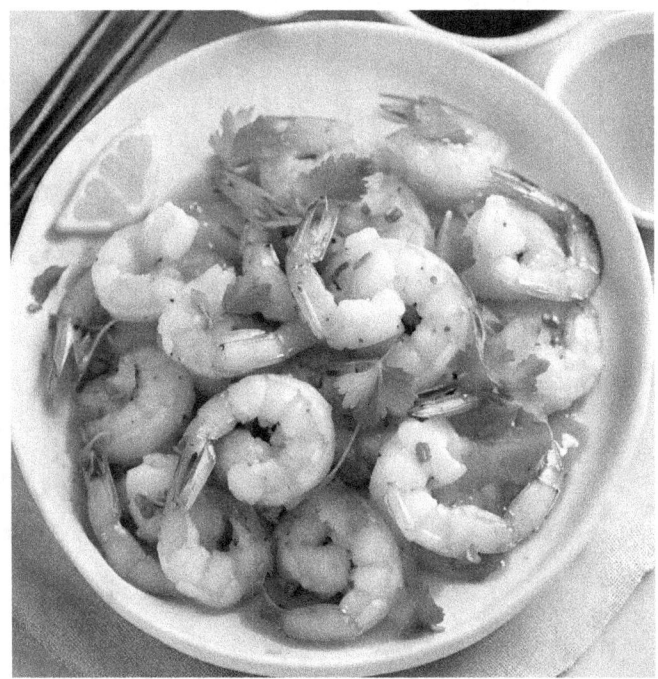

22. Calamari with Lemon and Parsley

Ingredients
- 1 pound calamari, cleaned and sliced into rings
- 2 tablespoons olive oil
- 2 cloves garlic, minced
- 2 tablespoons fresh lemon juice
- 1 teaspoon lemon zest
- 1/4 cup fresh parsley, chopped
- Lemon wedges for serving

Instructions
1. Heat olive oil in a large skillet over medium-high heat.
2. Add garlic and sauté for about 1 minute until fragrant.
3. Add calamari to the skillet and cook for 2-3 minutes, stirring frequently, until the calamari are opaque and cooked through.
4. Remove the skillet from heat and stir in lemon juice and lemon zest.
5. Sprinkle with fresh parsley.
6. Serve immediately with lemon wedges.

Nutrition Info per Serving
- Calories: 180
- Protein: 24g
- Carbohydrates: 3g
- Dietary Fiber: 1g
- Sugars: 0g
- Fat: 8g
- Saturated Fat: 1g
- Sodium: 160mg

Serves
4 servings
Cooking Time
10 minutes

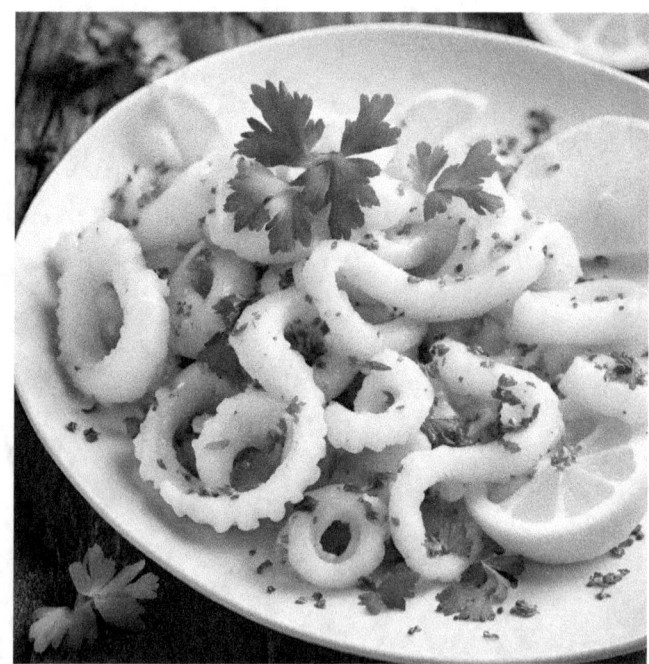

Poultry Recipes

1. Herb Roasted Chicken

Ingredients
- 1 whole chicken (about 4 pounds)
- 3 tablespoons olive oil
- 2 tablespoons fresh lemon juice
- 4 cloves garlic, minced
- 1 tablespoon fresh rosemary, chopped
- 1 tablespoon fresh thyme, chopped
- 1 tablespoon fresh parsley, chopped
- 1 teaspoon paprika
- 1 teaspoon garlic powder
- 1 teaspoon onion powder
- Lemon wedges for serving

Instructions
1. Preheat the oven to 375°F (190°C).
2. In a small bowl, mix together olive oil, lemon juice, garlic, rosemary, thyme, parsley, paprika, garlic powder, and onion powder.
3. Rinse the chicken and pat it dry with paper towels.
4. Rub the herb mixture all over the chicken, including under the skin.
5. Place the chicken in a roasting pan and roast for 1 hour and 20 minutes, or until the internal temperature reaches 165°F (75°C).
6. Let the chicken rest for 10 minutes before carving.
7. Serve with lemon wedges.

Nutrition Info per Serving
- Calories: 300
- Protein: 25g
- Carbohydrates: 2g
- Dietary Fiber: 1g
- Sugars: 0g
- Fat: 21g
- Saturated Fat: 5g
- Sodium: 85mg

Serves
6 servings

Cooking Time
1 hour 30 minutes

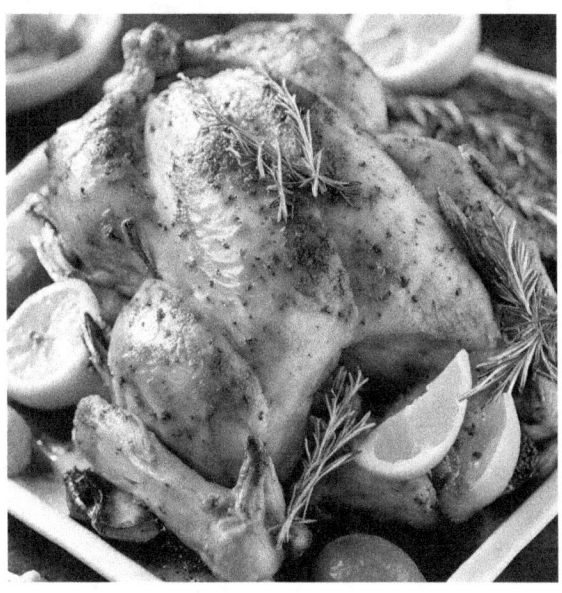

2. Lemon Garlic Turkey Breast

Ingredients
- 1 boneless, skinless turkey breast (about 2 pounds)
- 3 tablespoons olive oil
- 3 tablespoons fresh lemon juice
- 4 cloves garlic, minced
- 1 tablespoon fresh thyme, chopped
- 1 teaspoon paprika
- 1 teaspoon onion powder
- Lemon wedges for serving

Instructions
1. Preheat the oven to 375°F (190°C).
2. In a small bowl, mix together olive oil, lemon juice, garlic, thyme, paprika, and onion powder.
3. Rub the mixture all over the turkey breast.
4. Place the turkey breast in a baking dish and roast for 45-55 minutes, or until the internal temperature reaches 165°F (75°C).
5. Let the turkey rest for 10 minutes before slicing.
6. Serve with lemon wedges.

Nutrition Info per Serving
- Calories: 220
- Protein: 32g
- Carbohydrates: 2g
- Dietary Fiber: 0g
- Sugars: 0g
- Fat: 9g
- Saturated Fat: 1.5g
- Sodium: 70mg

Serves
6 servings
Cooking Time
55 minutes

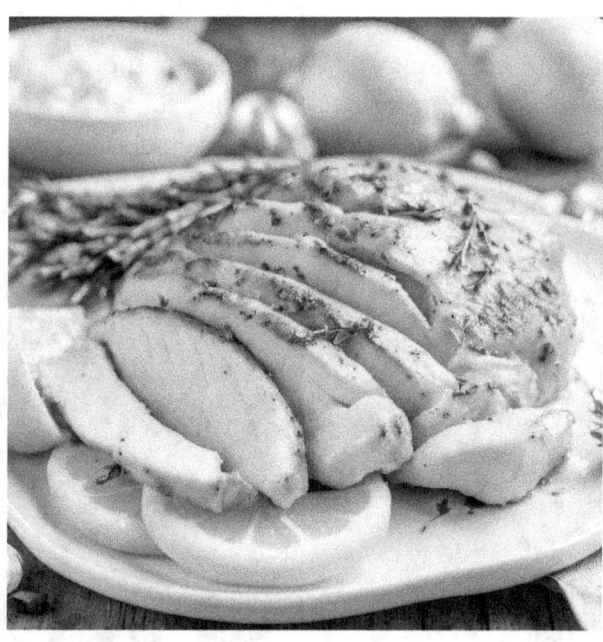

3. Balsamic Glazed Chicken

Ingredients
- 4 boneless, skinless chicken breasts (about 6 ounces each)
- 2 tablespoons olive oil
- 1/4 cup balsamic vinegar
- 2 tablespoons honey
- 2 cloves garlic, minced
- 1 teaspoon dried rosemary
- 1 teaspoon dried thyme

Instructions
1. Preheat the oven to 375°F (190°C).
2. In a small bowl, mix together balsamic vinegar, honey, garlic, rosemary, and thyme.
3. Heat olive oil in an oven-safe skillet over medium-high heat.
4. Add chicken breasts to the skillet and cook for 2-3 minutes on each side until browned.
5. Pour the balsamic mixture over the chicken.
6. Transfer the skillet to the oven and bake for 20-25 minutes, or until the internal temperature reaches 165°F (75°C).
7. Let the chicken rest for 5 minutes before serving.

Nutrition Info per Serving
- Calories: 250
- Protein: 32g
- Carbohydrates: 10g
- Dietary Fiber: 0g
- Sugars: 9g
- Fat: 9g
- Saturated Fat: 1.5g
- Sodium: 75mg

Serves
4 servings
Cooking Time
30 minutes

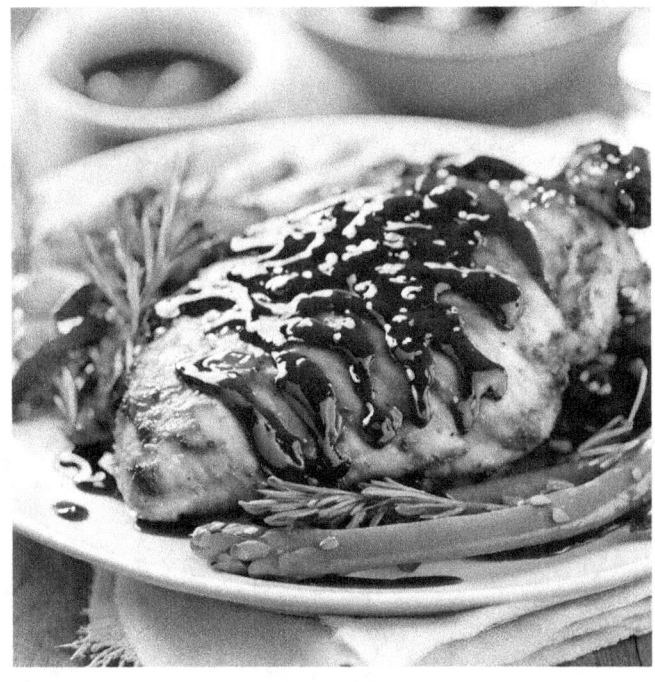

4. Spiced Roast Turkey

Ingredients
- 1 whole turkey (about 10 pounds)
- 4 tablespoons olive oil
- 2 tablespoons fresh lemon juice
- 4 cloves garlic, minced
- 1 tablespoon ground cumin
- 1 tablespoon ground paprika
- 1 teaspoon ground coriander
- 1 teaspoon ground cinnamon
- 1 teaspoon ground ginger
- Lemon wedges for serving

Instructions
1. Preheat the oven to 325°F (165°C).
2. In a small bowl, mix together olive oil, lemon juice, garlic, cumin, paprika, coriander, cinnamon, and ginger.
3. Rinse the turkey and pat it dry with paper towels.
4. Rub the spice mixture all over the turkey, including under the skin.
5. Place the turkey on a rack in a roasting pan and roast for 3 to 3 1/2 hours, or until the internal temperature reaches 165°F (75°C).
6. Let the turkey rest for 20 minutes before carving.
7. Serve with lemon wedges.

Nutrition Info per Serving
- Calories: 350
- Protein: 45g
- Carbohydrates: 3g
- Dietary Fiber: 1g
- Sugars: 1g
- Fat: 18g
- Saturated Fat: 5g
- Sodium: 90mg

Serves
12 servings

Cooking Time
3 hours 30 minutes

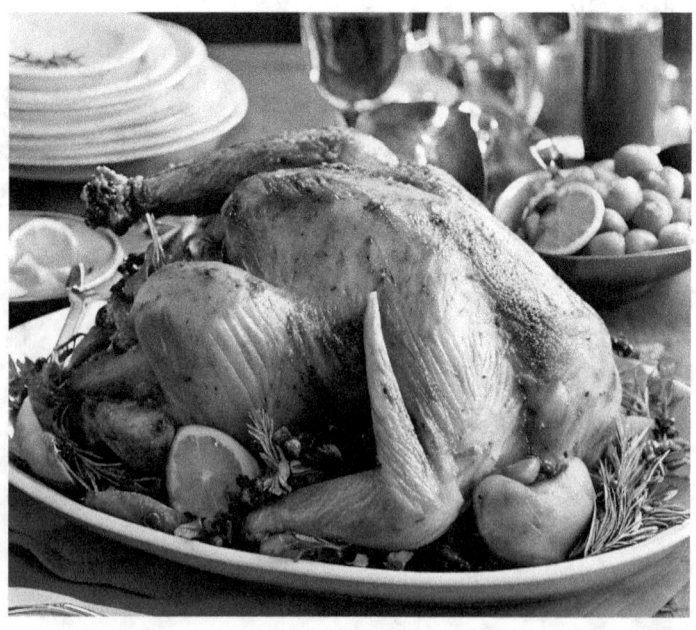

5. Apple Stuffed Chicken Breast

Ingredients
- 4 boneless, skinless chicken breasts (about 6 ounces each)
- 1 medium apple, peeled, cored, and diced
- 1/2 cup dried cranberries (unsweetened)
- 1/2 cup chopped walnuts (unsalted)
- 2 tablespoons olive oil
- 1 teaspoon dried thyme
- 1 teaspoon garlic powder
- 1 teaspoon onion powder
- 1 tablespoon fresh lemon juice

Instructions
1. Preheat the oven to 375°F (190°C).
2. In a bowl, combine diced apple, dried cranberries, and chopped walnuts.
3. Slice a pocket into each chicken breast, being careful not to cut all the way through.
4. Stuff each chicken breast with the apple mixture.
5. In a small bowl, mix olive oil, thyme, garlic powder, onion powder, and lemon juice.
6. Brush the olive oil mixture over the chicken breasts.
7. Place the chicken breasts in a baking dish and bake for 25-30 minutes, or until the internal temperature reaches 165°F (75°C).
8. Let the chicken rest for 5 minutes before serving.

Nutrition Info per Serving
- Calories: 300
- Protein: 32g
- Carbohydrates: 15g
- Dietary Fiber: 3g
- Sugars: 10g
- Fat: 13g
- Saturated Fat: 2g
- Sodium: 70mg

Serves
4 servings
Cooking Time
30 minutes

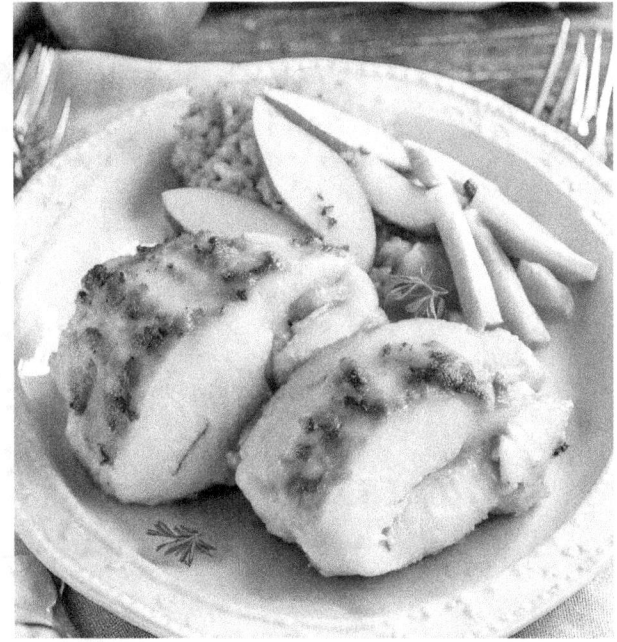

6. Mediterranean Turkey Meatloaf

Ingredients
- 1 pound ground turkey (lean)
- 1/2 cup rolled oats
- 1/4 cup low-sodium chicken broth
- 1/4 cup sun-dried tomatoes, chopped (no added salt)
- 1/4 cup crumbled feta cheese (low sodium)
- 1/4 cup fresh parsley, chopped
- 1/4 cup red onion, finely chopped
- 2 cloves garlic, minced
- 1 large egg
- 1 teaspoon dried oregano
- 1 teaspoon dried basil
- 1 tablespoon olive oil

Instructions
1. Preheat the oven to 375°F (190°C).
2. In a large bowl, combine ground turkey, rolled oats, chicken broth, sun-dried tomatoes, feta cheese, parsley, red onion, garlic, egg, oregano, and basil. Mix until well combined.
3. Transfer the mixture to a loaf pan and press it down evenly.
4. Brush the top with olive oil.
5. Bake for 45-50 minutes, or until the internal temperature reaches 165°F (75°C).
6. Let the meatloaf rest for 10 minutes before slicing and serving.

Nutrition Info per Serving
- Calories: 250
- Protein: 27g
- Carbohydrates: 10g
- Dietary Fiber: 2g
- Sugars: 3g
- Fat: 12g
- Saturated Fat: 3g
- Sodium: 150mg

Serves
4 servings

Cooking Time
50 minutes

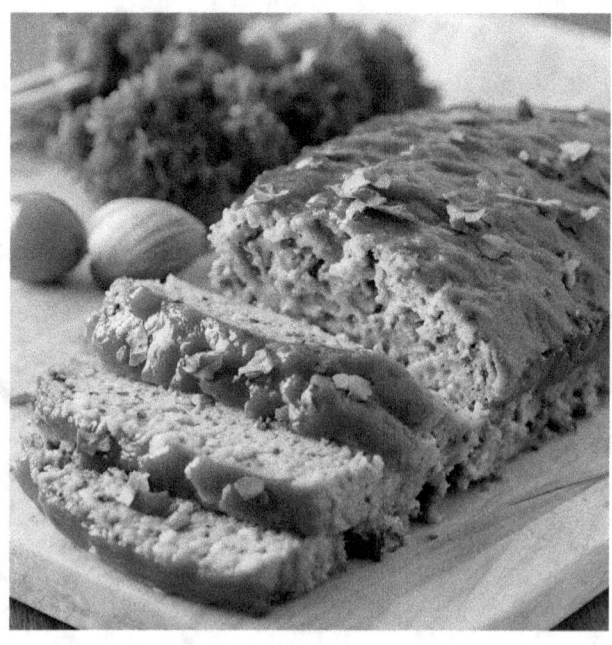

7. Pesto Rubbed Chicken

Ingredients
- 4 boneless, skinless chicken breasts (about 6 ounces each)
- 1/2 cup fresh basil leaves
- 1/4 cup pine nuts (unsalted)
- 2 cloves garlic
- 1/4 cup grated Parmesan cheese (low sodium or homemade)
- 1/4 cup olive oil
- 1 tablespoon fresh lemon juice

Instructions
1. Preheat the oven to 375°F (190°C).
2. In a food processor, combine basil leaves, pine nuts, garlic, Parmesan cheese, olive oil, and lemon juice. Blend until smooth to make the pesto.
3. Rub the pesto evenly over the chicken breasts.
4. Place the chicken breasts in a baking dish and bake for 25-30 minutes, or until the internal temperature reaches 165°F (75°C).
5. Let the chicken rest for 5 minutes before serving.

Nutrition Info per Serving
- Calories: 320
- Protein: 34g
- Carbohydrates: 2g
- Dietary Fiber: 1g
- Sugars: 0g
- Fat: 20g
- Saturated Fat: 4g
- Sodium: 140mg

Serves
4 servings
Cooking Time
30 minutes

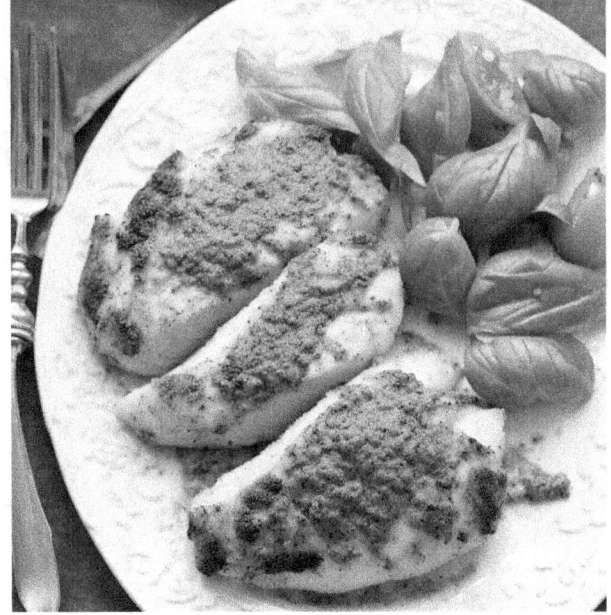

8. Orange Roast Chicken

Ingredients
- 1 whole chicken (about 4 pounds)
- 3 tablespoons olive oil
- 1/4 cup fresh orange juice
- 1 tablespoon orange zest
- 3 cloves garlic, minced
- 1 tablespoon fresh rosemary, chopped
- 1 tablespoon fresh thyme, chopped
- Orange slices for serving

Instructions
1. Preheat the oven to 375°F (190°C).
2. In a small bowl, mix together olive oil, orange juice, orange zest, garlic, rosemary, and thyme.
3. Rinse the chicken and pat it dry with paper towels.
4. Rub the orange mixture all over the chicken, including under the skin.
5. Place the chicken in a roasting pan and roast for 1 hour and 20 minutes, or until the internal temperature reaches 165°F (75°C).
6. Let the chicken rest for 10 minutes before carving.
7. Serve with orange slices.

Nutrition Info per Serving
- Calories: 320
- Protein: 28g
- Carbohydrates: 3g
- Dietary Fiber: 1g
- Sugars: 2g
- Fat: 21g
- Saturated Fat: 5g
- Sodium: 80mg

Serves
6 servings

Cooking Time
1 hour 30 minutes

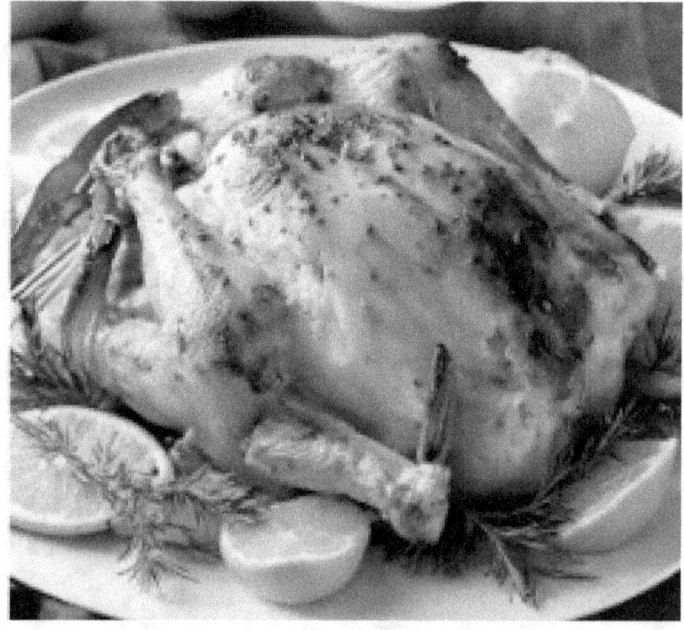

9. Grilled Chicken with Chimichurri

Ingredients
- 4 boneless, skinless chicken breasts (about 6 ounces each)
- 3 tablespoons olive oil
- 1/4 cup fresh parsley, chopped
- 1/4 cup fresh cilantro, chopped
- 2 cloves garlic, minced
- 2 tablespoons red wine vinegar
- 1 teaspoon dried oregano
- 1/4 teaspoon red pepper flakes
- 1 tablespoon fresh lemon juice

Instructions
1. Preheat the grill to medium-high heat.
2. In a bowl, mix together olive oil, parsley, cilantro, garlic, red wine vinegar, oregano, red pepper flakes, and lemon juice to make the chimichurri sauce.
3. Brush the chicken breasts with 1 tablespoon of the chimichurri sauce.
4. Grill the chicken breasts for 5-7 minutes on each side, or until the internal temperature reaches 165°F (75°C).
5. Let the chicken rest for 5 minutes before serving.
6. Serve the grilled chicken with the remaining chimichurri sauce on top.

Nutrition Info per Serving
- Calories: 280
- Protein: 34g
- Carbohydrates: 2g
- Dietary Fiber: 1g
- Sugars: 0g
- Fat: 15g
- Saturated Fat: 2.5g
- Sodium: 85mg

Serves
4 servings

Cooking Time
15 minutes

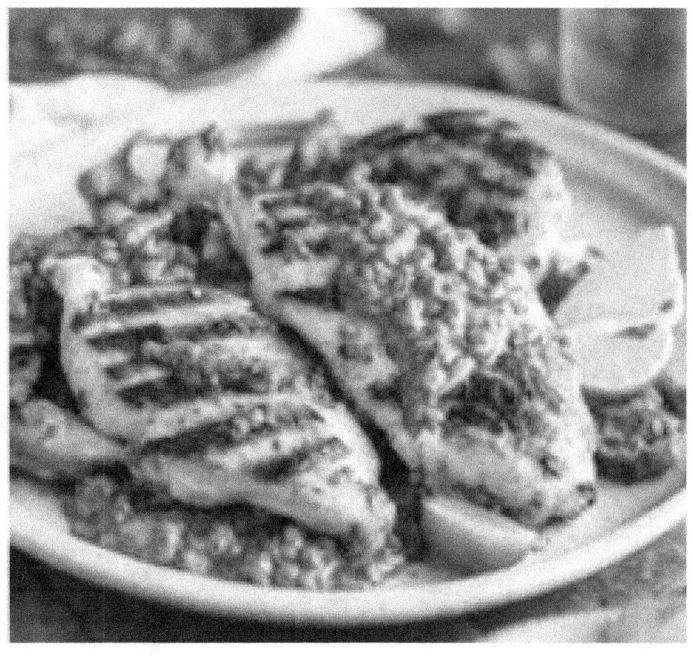

10. Turkey Burgers

Ingredients
- 1 pound ground turkey (lean)
- 1/4 cup finely chopped onion
- 2 cloves garlic, minced
- 1 tablespoon Dijon mustard (low sodium)
- 1 teaspoon dried oregano
- 1 teaspoon paprika
- 1 tablespoon olive oil (for grilling)
- Whole wheat buns (optional)
- Lettuce, tomato, and avocado slices (optional for serving)

Instructions
1. In a large bowl, combine ground turkey, onion, garlic, Dijon mustard, oregano, and paprika. Mix well.
2. Form the mixture into 4 equal patties.
3. Heat olive oil in a grill pan over medium-high heat.
4. Cook the turkey patties for 5-7 minutes on each side, or until the internal temperature reaches 165°F (75°C).
5. Serve on whole wheat buns with lettuce, tomato, and avocado slices if desired.

Nutrition Info per Serving
- Calories: 220
- Protein: 28g
- Carbohydrates: 4g
- Dietary Fiber: 1g
- Sugars: 1g
- Fat: 10g
- Saturated Fat: 2g
- Sodium: 120mg

Serves
4 servings

Cooking Time
15 minutes

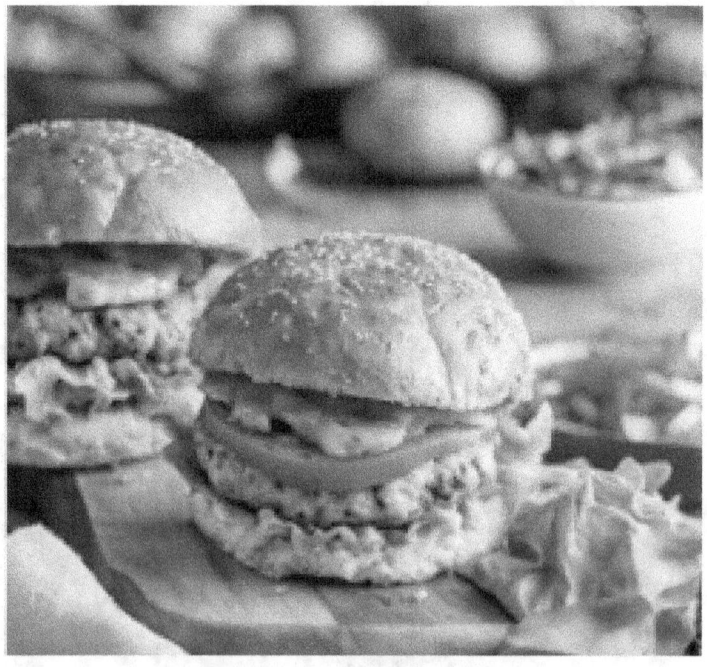

11. Grilled Turkey Steaks

Ingredients
- 4 turkey steaks (about 6 ounces each)
- 3 tablespoons olive oil
- 2 tablespoons fresh lemon juice
- 2 cloves garlic, minced
- 1 teaspoon dried thyme
- 1 teaspoon dried rosemary

Instructions
1. Preheat the grill to medium-high heat.
2. In a small bowl, mix together olive oil, lemon juice, garlic, thyme, and rosemary.
3. Brush the turkey steaks with the olive oil mixture.
4. Grill the turkey steaks for 5-7 minutes on each side, or until the internal temperature reaches 165°F (75°C).
5. Serve immediately.

Nutrition Info per Serving
- Calories: 240
- Protein: 34g
- Carbohydrates: 1g
- Dietary Fiber: 0g
- Sugars: 0g
- Fat: 10g
- Saturated Fat: 2g
- Sodium: 75mg

Serves
4 servings
Cooking Time
15 minutes

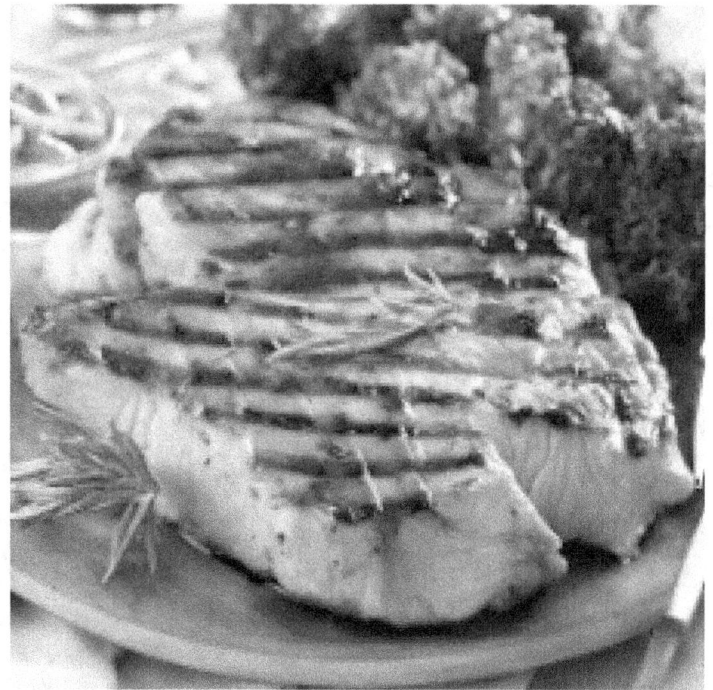

12. Barbecue Chicken

Ingredients
- 4 boneless, skinless chicken breasts (about 6 ounces each)
- 1/2 cup low-sodium barbecue sauce (store-bought or homemade)
- 1 tablespoon olive oil

Instructions
1. Preheat the grill to medium-high heat.
2. Brush the chicken breasts with olive oil.
3. Grill the chicken breasts for 5-7 minutes on each side, or until the internal temperature reaches 165°F (75°C).
4. During the last 2 minutes of grilling, brush the chicken breasts with barbecue sauce.
5. Serve immediately.

Nutrition Info per Serving
- Calories: 220
- Protein: 30g
- Carbohydrates: 10g
- Dietary Fiber: 1g
- Sugars: 8g
- Fat: 7g
- Saturated Fat: 1.5g
- Sodium: 150mg

Serves
4 servings
Cooking Time
15 minutes

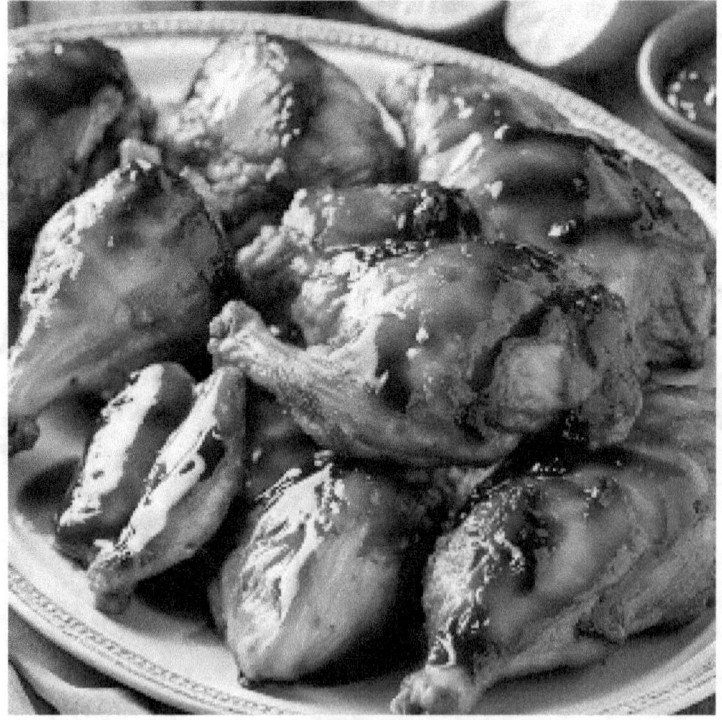

13. Broiled Turkey Cutlets with Dijon

Ingredients
- 4 turkey cutlets (about 6 ounces each)
- 3 tablespoons Dijon mustard (low sodium)
- 1 tablespoon honey
- 2 cloves garlic, minced
- 1 teaspoon dried thyme
- 1 tablespoon olive oil

Instructions
1. Preheat the broiler.
2. In a small bowl, mix together Dijon mustard, honey, garlic, thyme, and olive oil.
3. Brush the mustard mixture evenly over the turkey cutlets.
4. Place the turkey cutlets on a broiler pan and broil for 4-5 minutes on each side, or until the internal temperature reaches 165°F (75°C).
5. Serve immediately.

Nutrition Info per Serving
- Calories: 210
- Protein: 34g
- Carbohydrates: 5g
- Dietary Fiber: 0g
- Sugars: 4g
- Fat: 6g
- Saturated Fat: 1g
- Sodium: 140mg

Serves
4 servings
Cooking Time
10 minutes

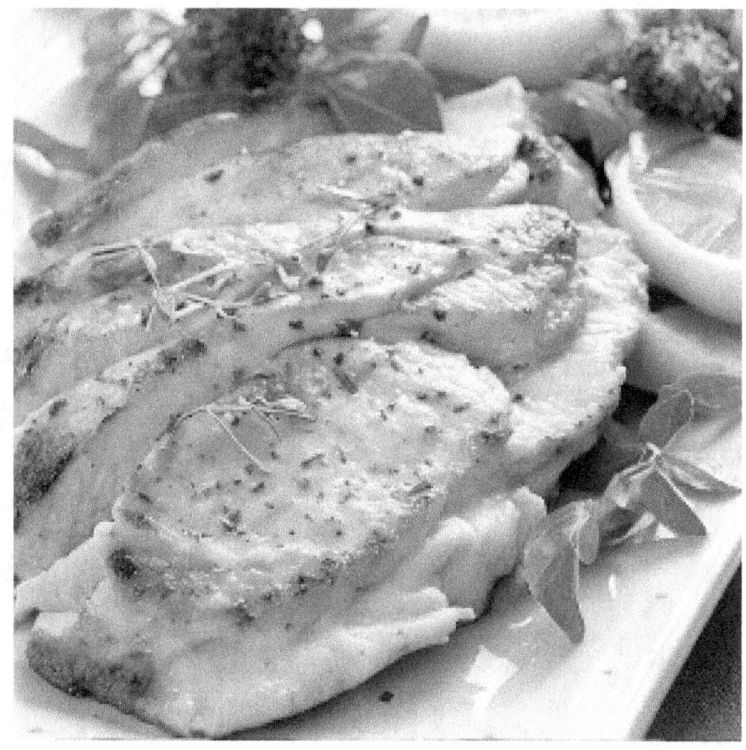

14. Tandoori Chicken

Ingredients
- 4 boneless, skinless chicken thighs (about 6 ounces each)
- 1 cup plain Greek yogurt (low-fat)
- 2 tablespoons fresh lemon juice
- 3 cloves garlic, minced
- 1 tablespoon grated fresh ginger
- 1 tablespoon ground cumin
- 1 tablespoon ground coriander
- 1 teaspoon ground turmeric
- 1 teaspoon paprika
- 1/2 teaspoon cayenne pepper (optional)

Instructions
1. In a large bowl, mix together Greek yogurt, lemon juice, garlic, ginger, cumin, coriander, turmeric, paprika, and cayenne pepper.
2. Add the chicken thighs to the marinade, coating them well. Cover and refrigerate for at least 2 hours, preferably overnight.
3. Preheat the grill to medium-high heat.
4. Remove the chicken from the marinade and shake off any excess.
5. Grill the chicken thighs for 5-7 minutes on each side, or until the internal temperature reaches 165°F (75°C).
6. Serve immediately.

Nutrition Info per Serving
- Calories: 250
- Protein: 32g
- Carbohydrates: 5g
- Dietary Fiber: 1g
- Sugars: 3g
- Fat: 11g
- Saturated Fat: 3g
- Sodium: 120mg

Serves
4 servings

Cooking Time
20 minutes (plus marinating time)

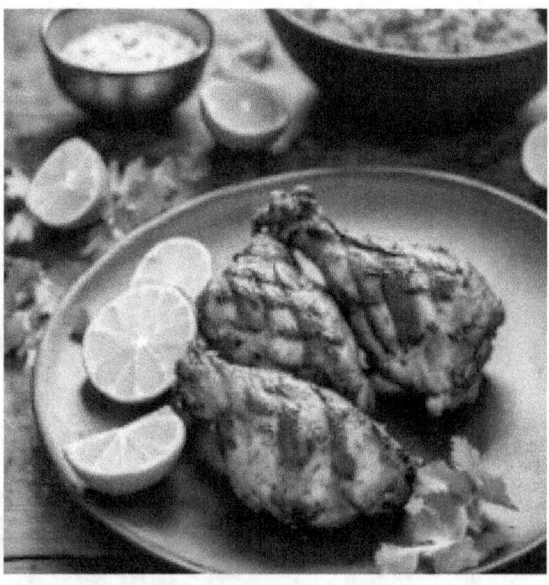

15. Thai Grilled Chicken

Ingredients
- 4 boneless, skinless chicken breasts (about 6 ounces each)
- 1/4 cup coconut milk (unsweetened)
- 2 tablespoons fresh lime juice
- 2 tablespoons low-sodium soy sauce
- 2 cloves garlic, minced
- 1 tablespoon grated fresh ginger
- 1 tablespoon honey
- 1 teaspoon ground coriander
- Fresh cilantro for garnish

Instructions
1. In a large bowl, mix together coconut milk, lime juice, soy sauce, garlic, ginger, honey, and ground coriander.
2. Add the chicken breasts to the marinade, coating them well. Cover and refrigerate for at least 1 hour.
3. Preheat the grill to medium-high heat.
4. Remove the chicken from the marinade and shake off any excess.
5. Grill the chicken breasts for 5-7 minutes on each side, or until the internal temperature reaches 165°F (75°C).
6. Garnish with fresh cilantro and serve immediately.

Nutrition Info per Serving
- Calories: 260
- Protein: 34g
- Carbohydrates: 6g
- Dietary Fiber: 1g
- Sugars: 5g
- Fat: 10g
- Saturated Fat: 3g
- Sodium: 140mg

Serves

4 servings

Cooking Time

15 minutes (plus marinating time)

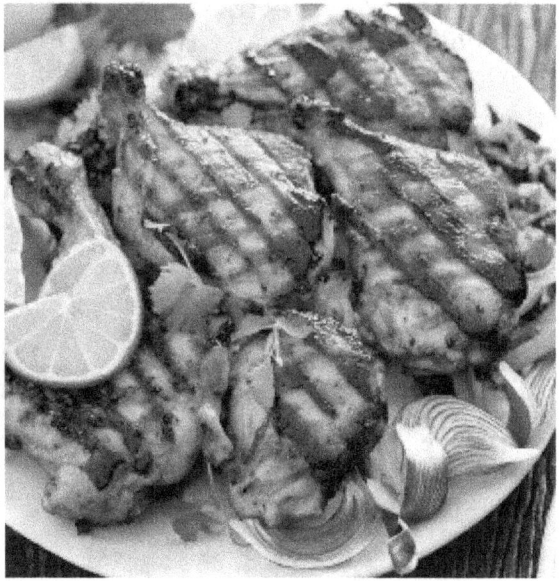

16. Turkey and White Bean Chili

Ingredients
- 1 pound ground turkey (lean)
- 2 tablespoons olive oil
- 1 large onion, diced
- 3 cloves garlic, minced
- 1 red bell pepper, diced
- 1 green bell pepper, diced
- 1 can (15 ounces) no-salt-added white beans, drained and rinsed
- 1 can (15 ounces) no-salt-added diced tomatoes
- 1 cup low-sodium chicken broth
- 2 tablespoons chili powder
- 1 teaspoon ground cumin
- 1 teaspoon smoked paprika
- 1/2 teaspoon dried oregano
- 1/2 teaspoon cayenne pepper (optional)
- Fresh cilantro for garnish (optional)

Instructions
1. Heat olive oil in a large pot over medium heat. Add onion and garlic, and sauté until softened, about 5 minutes.
2. Add ground turkey and cook until browned, breaking it up with a spoon, about 7-8 minutes.
3. Add red bell pepper and green bell pepper, and cook for another 5 minutes.
4. Stir in chili powder, cumin, smoked paprika, oregano, and cayenne pepper (if using). Cook for 1-2 minutes until fragrant.
5. Add white beans, diced tomatoes, and chicken broth. Stir well to combine.
6. Bring to a boil, then reduce heat and simmer for 30 minutes, stirring occasionally.
7. Serve hot, garnished with fresh cilantro if desired.

Nutrition Info per Serving
- Calories: 280
- Protein: 25g
- Carbohydrates: 25g
- Dietary Fiber: 7g
- Sugars: 6g
- Fat: 10g
- Saturated Fat: 2g
- Sodium: 150mg

Serves
6 servings
Cooking Time
50 minutes

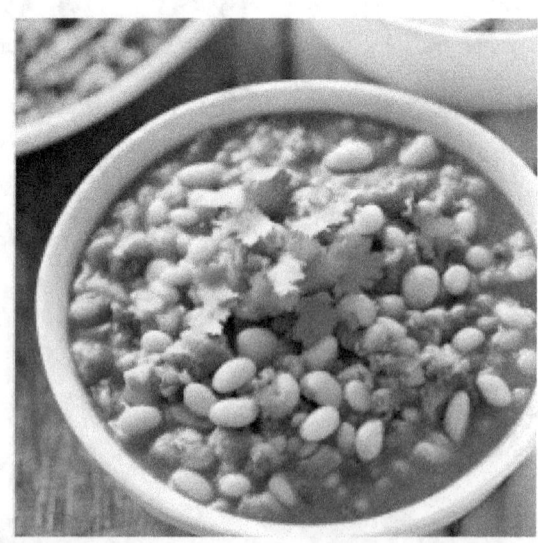

17. Lemon Chicken Orzo Soup

Ingredients
- 1 pound boneless, skinless chicken breasts, diced
- 2 tablespoons olive oil
- 1 large onion, diced
- 3 cloves garlic, minced
- 2 medium carrots, diced
- 2 celery stalks, diced
- 6 cups low-sodium chicken broth
- 1 cup uncooked orzo pasta
- 1/4 cup fresh lemon juice
- 2 teaspoons lemon zest
- 1 teaspoon dried thyme
- 1 teaspoon dried basil
- 1 cup fresh spinach, chopped
- Fresh parsley for garnish (optional)

Instructions
1. Heat olive oil in a large pot over medium heat. Add onion and garlic, and sauté until softened, about 5 minutes.
2. Add diced chicken and cook until browned, about 5-7 minutes.
3. Add carrots and celery, and cook for another 5 minutes.
4. Stir in chicken broth, lemon juice, lemon zest, thyme, and basil. Bring to a boil.
5. Add orzo pasta and reduce heat to a simmer. Cook until orzo is tender, about 10-12 minutes.
6. Stir in fresh spinach and cook until wilted, about 2 minutes.
7. Serve hot, garnished with fresh parsley if desired.

Nutrition Info per Serving
- Calories: 250
- Protein: 28g
- Carbohydrates: 28g
- Dietary Fiber: 3g
- Sugars: 5g
- Fat: 6g
- Saturated Fat: 1g
- Sodium: 150mg

Serves
6 servings
Cooking Time
40 minutes

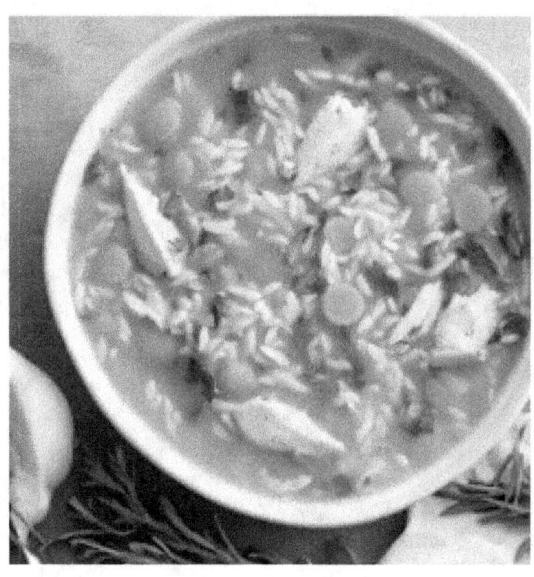

18. Creamy Turkey and Wild Rice Soup

Ingredients
- 1 pound cooked turkey breast, diced
- 2 tablespoons olive oil
- 1 large onion, diced
- 3 cloves garlic, minced
- 2 medium carrots, diced
- 2 celery stalks, diced
- 1 cup uncooked wild rice
- 6 cups low-sodium chicken broth
- 1 cup low-fat milk
- 1/2 cup plain Greek yogurt (low-fat)
- 1 teaspoon dried thyme
- 1 teaspoon dried rosemary
- Fresh parsley for garnish (optional)

Instructions
1. Heat olive oil in a large pot over medium heat. Add onion and garlic, and sauté until softened, about 5 minutes.
2. Add carrots and celery, and cook for another 5 minutes.
3. Stir in wild rice and cook for 1-2 minutes to lightly toast the rice.
4. Add chicken broth, thyme, and rosemary. Bring to a boil, then reduce heat to a simmer and cook until the rice is tender, about 45 minutes.
5. Stir in diced turkey and cook until heated through, about 5 minutes.
6. In a small bowl, whisk together milk and Greek yogurt until smooth. Stir the mixture into the soup and cook for another 5 minutes until creamy.
7. Serve hot, garnished with fresh parsley if desired.

Nutrition Info per Serving
- Calories: 280
- Protein: 28g
- Carbohydrates: 32g
- Dietary Fiber: 4g
- Sugars: 5g
- Fat: 8g
- Saturated Fat: 2g
- Sodium: 160mg

Serves
6 servings

Cooking Time
1 hour

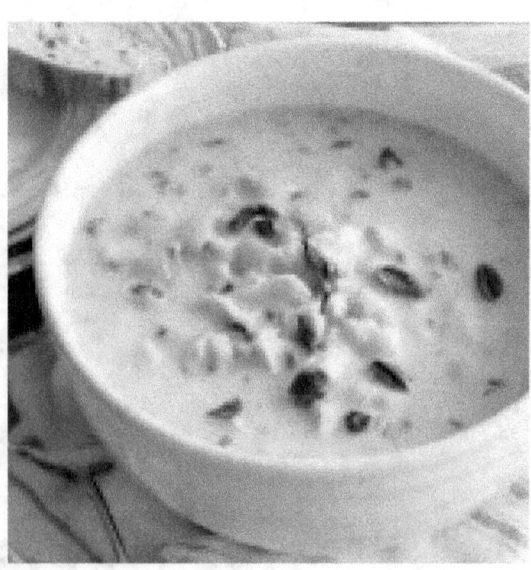

19. Chicken Piccata

Ingredients
- 4 boneless, skinless chicken breasts (about 6 ounces each)
- 1/4 cup whole wheat flour
- 3 tablespoons olive oil
- 1/4 cup fresh lemon juice
- 1/4 cup low-sodium chicken broth
- 1/4 cup capers, rinsed and drained
- 2 cloves garlic, minced
- 1 tablespoon fresh parsley, chopped
- Lemon slices for garnish

Instructions
1. Place the chicken breasts between two pieces of plastic wrap and pound to an even thickness.
2. Dredge the chicken breasts in whole wheat flour, shaking off any excess.
3. Heat 2 tablespoons of olive oil in a large skillet over medium-high heat.
4. Cook the chicken breasts for 4-5 minutes on each side until golden brown and cooked through. Remove from the skillet and keep warm.
5. In the same skillet, add the remaining olive oil and garlic. Cook for about 1 minute until fragrant.
6. Add lemon juice, chicken broth, and capers. Bring to a boil and cook for 2-3 minutes until the sauce thickens slightly.
7. Return the chicken breasts to the skillet and simmer for another 2 minutes.
8. Serve the chicken with the sauce, garnished with fresh parsley and lemon slices.

Nutrition Info per Serving
- Calories: 300
- Protein: 34g
- Carbohydrates: 10g
- Dietary Fiber: 1g
- Sugars: 1g
- Fat: 14g
- Saturated Fat: 2.5g
- Sodium: 140mg

Serves
4 servings

Cooking Time
20 minutes

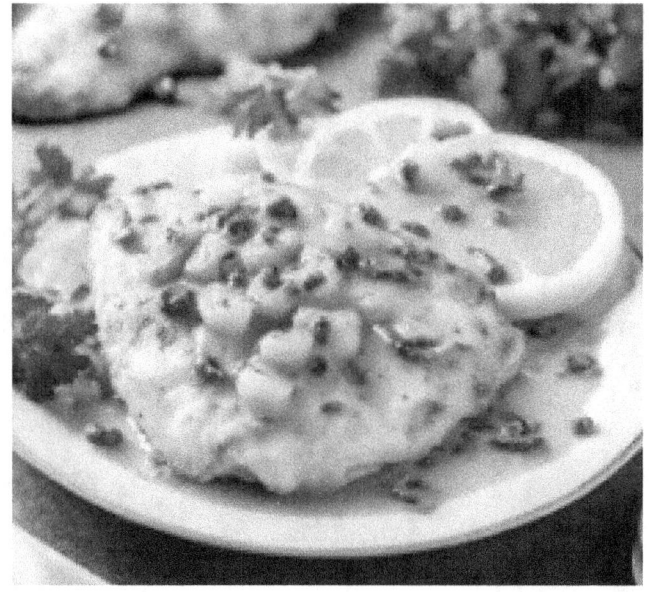

20. Turkey Scallopini

Ingredients
- 1 pound turkey cutlets
- 1/4 cup whole wheat flour
- 3 tablespoons olive oil
- 1/4 cup dry white wine
- 1/4 cup low-sodium chicken broth
- 2 cloves garlic, minced
- 1 tablespoon fresh lemon juice
- 1 tablespoon fresh parsley, chopped

Instructions
1. Dredge the turkey cutlets in whole wheat flour, shaking off any excess.
2. Heat 2 tablespoons of olive oil in a large skillet over medium-high heat.
3. Cook the turkey cutlets for 2-3 minutes on each side until golden brown and cooked through. Remove from the skillet and keep warm.
4. In the same skillet, add the remaining olive oil and garlic. Cook for about 1 minute until fragrant.
5. Add white wine and chicken broth. Bring to a boil and cook for 2-3 minutes until the sauce reduces slightly.
6. Stir in lemon juice.
7. Return the turkey cutlets to the skillet and simmer for another 2 minutes.
8. Serve the turkey with the sauce, garnished with fresh parsley.

Nutrition Info per Serving
- Calories: 260
- Protein: 30g
- Carbohydrates: 8g
- Dietary Fiber: 1g
- Sugars: 1g
- Fat: 12g
- Saturated Fat: 2.5g
- Sodium: 110mg

Serves
4 servings

Cooking Time
20 minutes

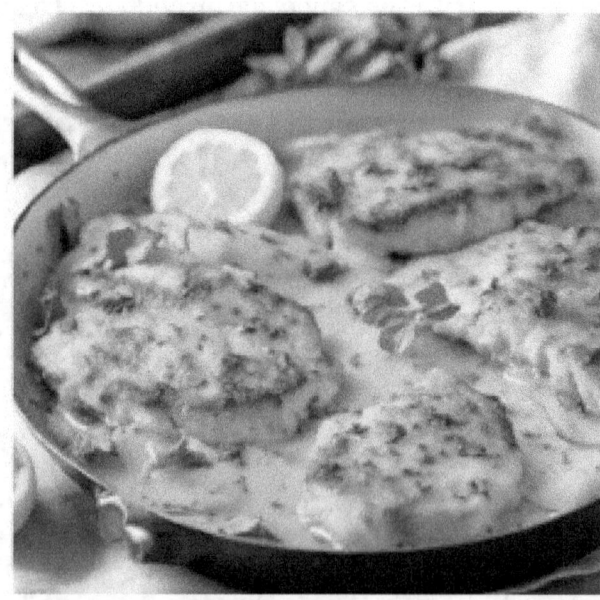

21. Stir-Fried Turkey with Vegetables

Ingredients
- 1 pound turkey breast, thinly sliced
- 2 tablespoons olive oil
- 1 large onion, sliced
- 2 cloves garlic, minced
- 1 red bell pepper, sliced
- 1 yellow bell pepper, sliced
- 1 cup broccoli florets
- 1/2 cup carrots, julienned
- 1/4 cup low-sodium soy sauce
- 1 tablespoon fresh ginger, grated
- 1 tablespoon honey
- 1 tablespoon rice vinegar
- 1 teaspoon cornstarch mixed with 1 tablespoon water (optional for thickening)

Instructions
1. Heat 1 tablespoon of olive oil in a large skillet or wok over medium-high heat.
2. Add the turkey slices and stir-fry until browned and cooked through, about 5-7 minutes. Remove from the skillet and keep warm.
3. In the same skillet, heat the remaining olive oil. Add onion and garlic, and stir-fry for 2-3 minutes until fragrant.
4. Add bell peppers, broccoli, and carrots. Stir-fry for 5-7 minutes until the vegetables are tender-crisp.
5. In a small bowl, mix together soy sauce, ginger, honey, and rice vinegar. Add the sauce to the skillet.
6. Return the turkey to the skillet and stir to combine. If a thicker sauce is desired, add the cornstarch mixture and cook for an additional 1-2 minutes.
7. Serve immediately.

Nutrition Info per Serving
- Calories: 250
- Protein: 28g
- Carbohydrates: 15g
- Dietary Fiber: 3g
- Sugars: 7g
- Fat: 10g
- Saturated Fat: 1.5g
- Sodium: 150mg

Serves
4 servings

Cooking Time
20 minutes

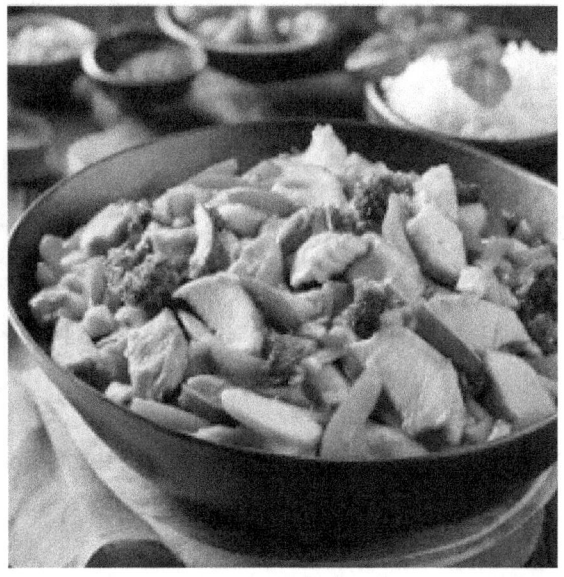

22. Pan-Seared Chicken with Spinach

Ingredients
- 4 boneless, skinless chicken breasts (about 6 ounces each)
- 2 tablespoons olive oil
- 3 cloves garlic, minced
- 1/4 cup low-sodium chicken broth
- 1 tablespoon fresh lemon juice
- 1 teaspoon dried thyme
- 4 cups fresh spinach leaves
- Lemon wedges for serving

Instructions
1. Heat 1 tablespoon of olive oil in a large skillet over medium-high heat.
2. Cook the chicken breasts for 5-7 minutes on each side until golden brown and cooked through. Remove from the skillet and keep warm.
3. In the same skillet, heat the remaining olive oil. Add garlic and cook for about 1 minute until fragrant.
4. Add chicken broth, lemon juice, and thyme. Bring to a boil and cook for 2-3 minutes until the sauce reduces slightly.
5. Add spinach to the skillet and cook until wilted, about 2 minutes.
6. Return the chicken breasts to the skillet and simmer for another 2 minutes.
7. Serve the chicken with the spinach and sauce, garnished with lemon wedges.

Nutrition Info per Serving
- Calories: 260
- Protein: 34g
- Carbohydrates: 4g
- Dietary Fiber: 2g
- Sugars: 1g
- Fat: 11g
- Saturated Fat: 2g
- Sodium: 120mg

Serves
4 servings

Cooking Time
20 minutes

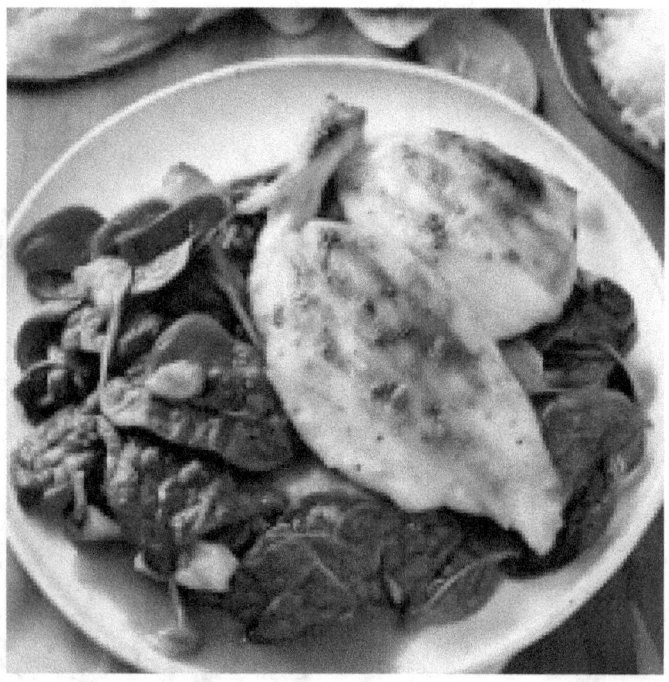

23. Chicken Marsala

Ingredients
- 4 boneless, skinless chicken breasts (about 6 ounces each)
- 1/4 cup whole wheat flour
- 3 tablespoons olive oil
- 1/2 cup dry Marsala wine
- 1/2 cup low-sodium chicken broth
- 1 cup mushrooms, sliced
- 2 cloves garlic, minced
- 1 teaspoon dried oregano
- Fresh parsley for garnish (optional)

Instructions
1. Place the chicken breasts between two pieces of plastic wrap and pound to an even thickness.
2. Dredge the chicken breasts in whole wheat flour, shaking off any excess.
3. Heat 2 tablespoons of olive oil in a large skillet over medium-high heat.
4. Cook the chicken breasts for 4-5 minutes on each side until golden brown and cooked through. Remove from the skillet and keep warm.
5. In the same skillet, add the remaining olive oil and garlic. Cook for about 1 minute until fragrant.
6. Add mushrooms and cook for 3-4 minutes until they begin to brown.
7. Stir in Marsala wine and chicken broth. Bring to a boil and cook for 2-3 minutes until the sauce thickens slightly.
8. Return the chicken breasts to the skillet and simmer for another 2 minutes.
9. Serve the chicken with the sauce, garnished with fresh parsley if desired.

Nutrition Info per Serving
- Calories: 310
- Protein: 34g
- Carbohydrates: 10g
- Dietary Fiber: 1g
- Sugars: 2g
- Fat: 14g
- Saturated Fat: 2.5g
- Sodium: 140mg

Serves
4 servings

Cooking Time
25 minutes

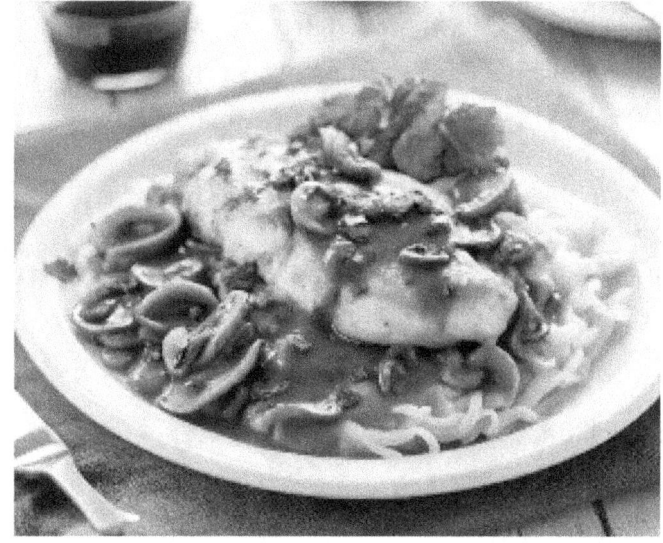

Soups & Salads

1. Garden Vegetable Soup
Ingredients
- 2 tablespoons olive oil
- 1 large onion, diced
- 3 cloves garlic, minced
- 2 medium carrots, diced
- 2 celery stalks, diced
- 1 zucchini, diced
- 1 yellow squash, diced
- 1 bell pepper, diced
- 1 cup green beans, trimmed and cut into 1-inch pieces
- 4 cups low-sodium vegetable broth
- 1 can (15 ounces) no-salt-added diced tomatoes
- 1 teaspoon dried thyme
- 1 teaspoon dried basil
- 1/2 teaspoon dried oregano
- 1/4 teaspoon cayenne pepper (optional)
- 1 cup kale, chopped
- Fresh parsley for garnish

Instructions
1. Heat olive oil in a large pot over medium heat. Add onion and garlic, and sauté until softened, about 5 minutes.
2. Add carrots and celery, and cook for another 5 minutes.
3. Stir in zucchini, yellow squash, bell pepper, and green beans. Cook for 5 minutes.
4. Add vegetable broth, diced tomatoes, thyme, basil, oregano, and cayenne pepper (if using). Bring to a boil, then reduce heat and simmer for 20 minutes.
5. Stir in kale and cook for another 5 minutes.
6. Serve hot, garnished with fresh parsley.

Nutrition Info per Serving
- Calories: 120 Protein: 3g Carbohydrates: 20g Dietary Fiber: 5g
- Sugars: 8g
- Fat: 4g
- Saturated Fat: 0.5g
- Sodium: 120mg

Serves
6 servings
Cooking Time
40 minutes

2. Pumpkin Soup

Ingredients
- 2 tablespoons olive oil
- 1 large onion, diced
- 3 cloves garlic, minced
- 1 can (15 ounces) pumpkin puree (no added salt)
- 4 cups low-sodium vegetable broth
- 1 cup unsweetened almond milk
- 1 teaspoon ground cumin
- 1 teaspoon ground cinnamon
- 1/2 teaspoon ground nutmeg
- 1/4 teaspoon ground ginger
- Fresh parsley for garnish

Instructions
1. Heat olive oil in a large pot over medium heat. Add onion and garlic, and sauté until softened, about 5 minutes.
2. Stir in pumpkin puree, vegetable broth, almond milk, cumin, cinnamon, nutmeg, and ginger. Bring to a boil.
3. Reduce heat and simmer for 20 minutes, stirring occasionally.
4. Use an immersion blender to puree the soup until smooth.
5. Serve hot, garnished with fresh parsley.

Nutrition Info per Serving
- Calories: 150
- Protein: 3g
- Carbohydrates: 20g
- Dietary Fiber: 5g
- Sugars: 7g
- Fat: 6g
- Saturated Fat: 1g
- Sodium: 110mg

Serves
4 servings
Cooking Time
30 minutes

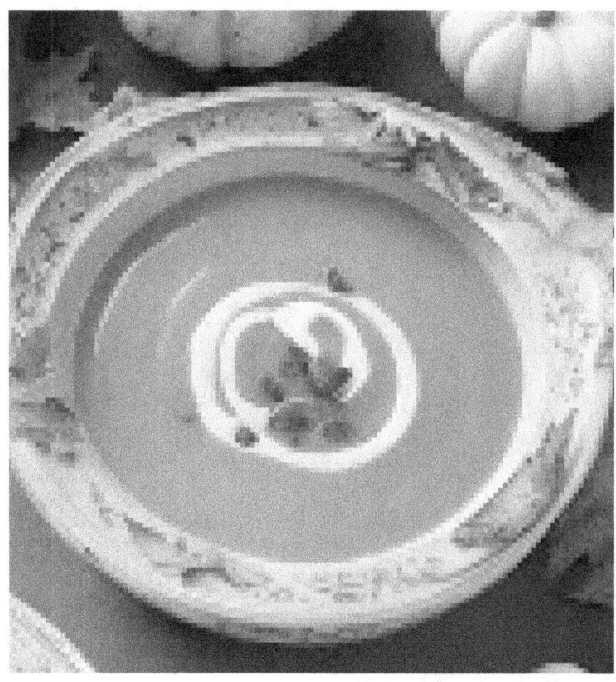

3. Mixed Greens with Apple Slices

Ingredients
- 6 cups mixed salad greens (such as spinach, arugula, and kale)
- 1 large apple, thinly sliced
- 1/4 cup walnuts, chopped (unsalted)
- 1/4 cup dried cranberries (unsweetened)
- 2 tablespoons olive oil
- 1 tablespoon apple cider vinegar
- 1 teaspoon Dijon mustard (low sodium)
- 1 teaspoon honey

Instructions
1. In a large bowl, combine mixed greens, apple slices, walnuts, and dried cranberries.
2. In a small bowl, whisk together olive oil, apple cider vinegar, Dijon mustard, and honey.
3. Drizzle the dressing over the salad and toss to combine.
4. Serve immediately.

Nutrition Info per Serving
- Calories: 180
- Protein: 2g
- Carbohydrates: 18g
- Dietary Fiber: 4g
- Sugars: 12g
- Fat: 12g
- Saturated Fat: 1.5g
- Sodium: 60mg

Serves
4 servings
Cooking Time
10 minutes

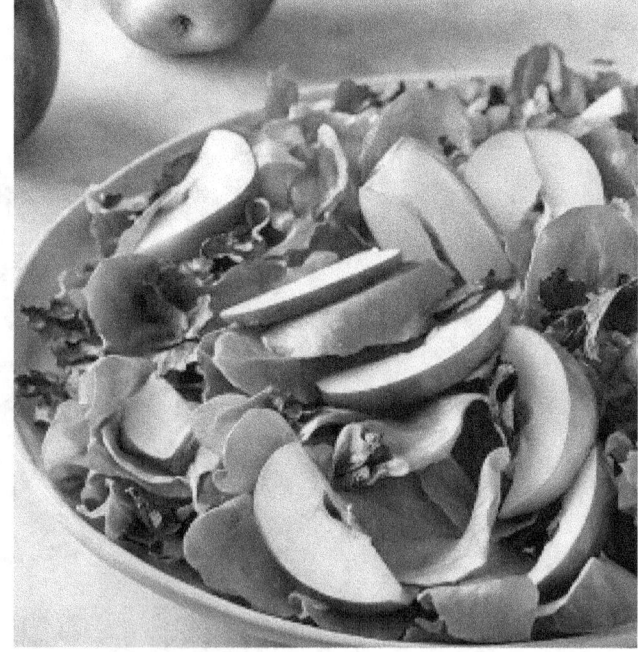

4. Beet and Goat Cheese Salad

Ingredients
- 4 medium beets, roasted and sliced
- 6 cups mixed salad greens (such as spinach, arugula, and kale)
- 1/4 cup goat cheese, crumbled (low sodium)
- 1/4 cup walnuts, chopped (unsalted)
- 2 tablespoons balsamic vinegar
- 2 tablespoons olive oil
- 1 teaspoon Dijon mustard (low sodium)
- 1 teaspoon honey

Instructions
1. Preheat the oven to 400°F (200°C). Wrap the beets in aluminum foil and roast for 45-60 minutes until tender. Let cool, then peel and slice.
2. In a large bowl, combine mixed greens, roasted beets, goat cheese, and walnuts.
3. In a small bowl, whisk together balsamic vinegar, olive oil, Dijon mustard, and honey.
4. Drizzle the dressing over the salad and toss to combine.
5. Serve immediately.

Nutrition Info per Serving
- Calories: 220
- Protein: 4g
- Carbohydrates: 18g
- Dietary Fiber: 5g
- Sugars: 10g
- Fat: 15g
- Saturated Fat: 4g
- Sodium: 90mg

Serves
4 servings

Cooking Time
1 hour

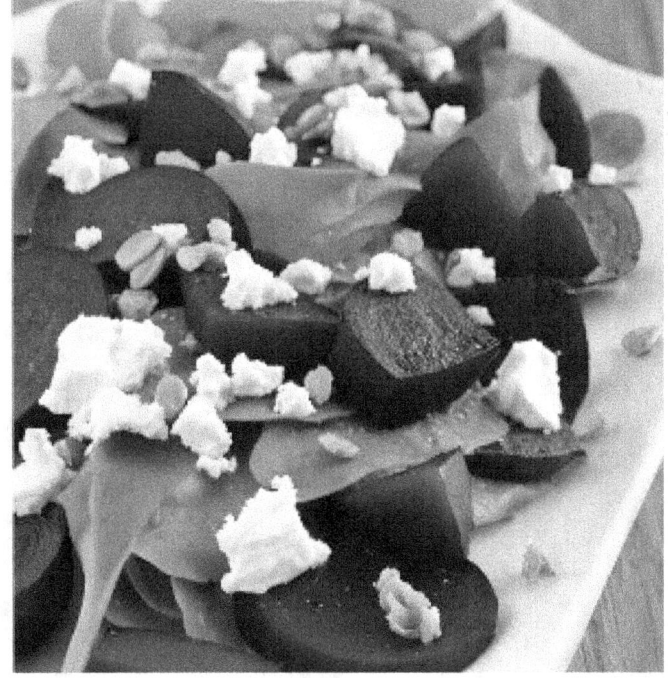

5. Barley and Mushroom Soup

Ingredients
- 2 tablespoons olive oil
- 1 large onion, diced
- 3 cloves garlic, minced
- 2 cups mushrooms, sliced
- 1 cup pearl barley, rinsed
- 4 cups low-sodium vegetable broth
- 1 cup water
- 2 carrots, diced
- 2 celery stalks, diced
- 1 teaspoon dried thyme
- 1 teaspoon dried rosemary
- Fresh parsley for garnish

Instructions
1. Heat olive oil in a large pot over medium heat. Add onion and garlic, and sauté until softened, about 5 minutes.
2. Add mushrooms and cook until they release their moisture and begin to brown, about 5-7 minutes.
3. Stir in barley, vegetable broth, water, carrots, celery, thyme, and rosemary. Bring to a boil.
4. Reduce heat and simmer for 40-45 minutes, or until the barley is tender.
5. Serve hot, garnished with fresh parsley.

Nutrition Info per Serving
- Calories: 220
- Protein: 5g
- Carbohydrates: 36g
- Dietary Fiber: 8g
- Sugars: 8g
- Fat: 7g
- Saturated Fat: 1g
- Sodium: 120mg

Serves
6 servings

Cooking Time
50 minutes

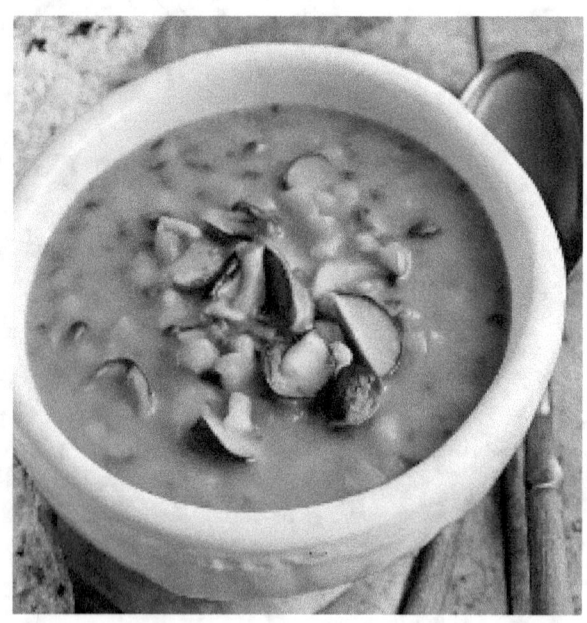

6. Split Pea Soup

Ingredients
- 2 tablespoons olive oil
- 1 large onion, diced
- 3 cloves garlic, minced
- 2 cups dried split peas, rinsed
- 6 cups low-sodium vegetable broth
- 2 carrots, diced
- 2 celery stalks, diced
- 1 teaspoon dried thyme
- 1 teaspoon dried marjoram
- 1 bay leaf
- Fresh parsley for garnish

Instructions
1. Heat olive oil in a large pot over medium heat. Add onion and garlic, and sauté until softened, about 5 minutes.
2. Add split peas, vegetable broth, carrots, celery, thyme, marjoram, and bay leaf. Bring to a boil.
3. Reduce heat and simmer for 60-70 minutes, or until the peas are tender and the soup is thickened.
4. Remove the bay leaf before serving.
5. Serve hot, garnished with fresh parsley.

Nutrition Info per Serving
- Calories: 250
- Protein: 16g
- Carbohydrates: 42g
- Dietary Fiber: 16g
- Sugars: 7g
- Fat: 5g
- Saturated Fat: 0.5g
- Sodium: 140mg

Serves
6 servings

Cooking Time
1 hour 15 minutes

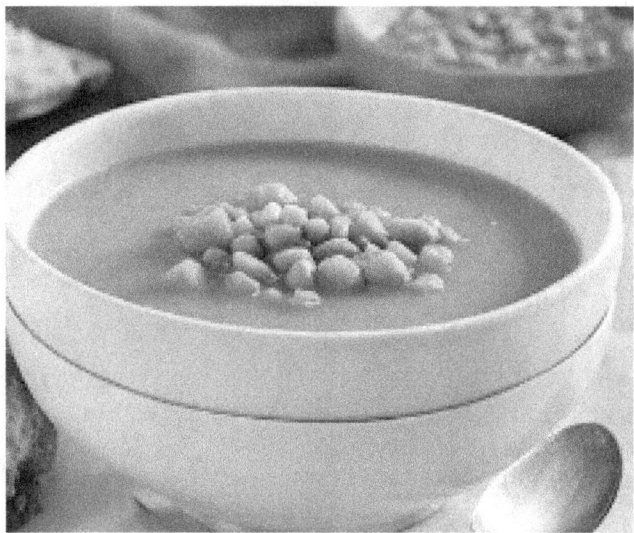

7. Beetroot and Ginger Soup

Ingredients
- 2 tablespoons olive oil
- 1 large onion, diced
- 3 cloves garlic, minced
- 1 tablespoon fresh ginger, grated
- 4 medium beetroots, peeled and diced
- 4 cups low-sodium vegetable broth
- 1 cup water
- 1 teaspoon ground cumin
- 1 teaspoon ground coriander
- Fresh dill for garnish

Instructions
1. Heat olive oil in a large pot over medium heat. Add onion, garlic, and ginger, and sauté until softened, about 5 minutes.
2. Add diced beetroot, vegetable broth, water, cumin, and coriander. Bring to a boil.
3. Reduce heat and simmer for 30-35 minutes, or until the beetroots are tender.
4. Use an immersion blender to puree the soup until smooth.
5. Serve hot, garnished with fresh dill.

Nutrition Info per Serving
- Calories: 160
- Protein: 3g
- Carbohydrates: 23g
- Dietary Fiber: 5g
- Sugars: 14g
- Fat: 7g
- Saturated Fat: 1g
- Sodium: 110mg

Serves
4 servings
Cooking Time
40 minutes

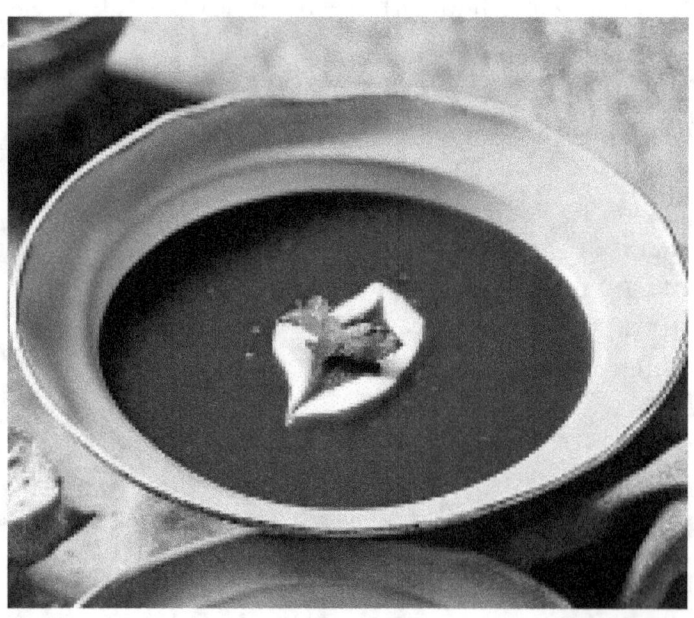

8. Carrot and Coriander Soup

Ingredients
- 2 tablespoons olive oil
- 1 large onion, diced
- 3 cloves garlic, minced
- 1 tablespoon ground coriander
- 6 large carrots, peeled and diced
- 4 cups low-sodium vegetable broth
- 1 cup water
- 1/4 cup fresh coriander leaves, chopped
- Fresh coriander leaves for garnish

Instructions
1. Heat olive oil in a large pot over medium heat. Add onion and garlic, and sauté until softened, about 5 minutes.
2. Stir in ground coriander and cook for another minute.
3. Add carrots, vegetable broth, and water. Bring to a boil.
4. Reduce heat and simmer for 25-30 minutes, or until the carrots are tender.
5. Use an immersion blender to puree the soup until smooth.
6. Stir in fresh coriander leaves.
7. Serve hot, garnished with additional fresh coriander leaves.

Nutrition Info per Serving
- Calories: 180
- Protein: 2g
- Carbohydrates: 24g
- Dietary Fiber: 6g
- Sugars: 12g
- Fat: 9g
- Saturated Fat: 1.5g
- Sodium: 100mg

Serves
4 servings
Cooking Time
35 minutes

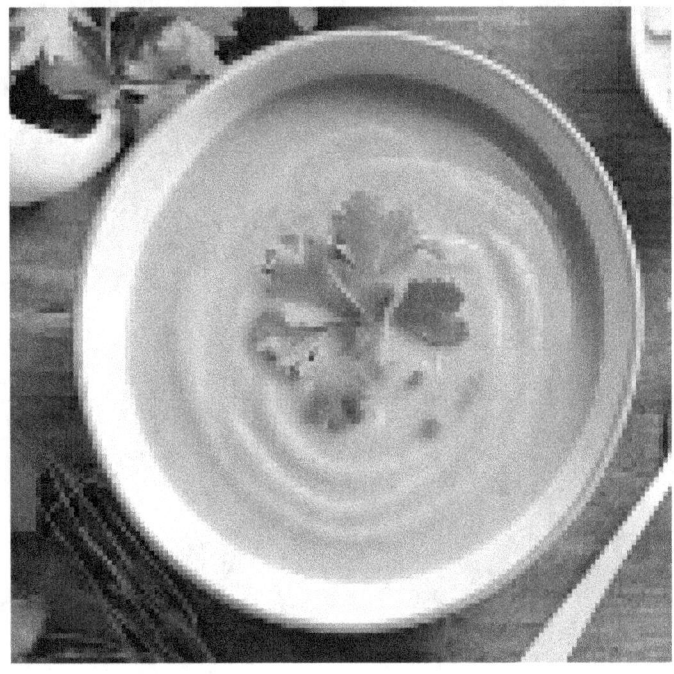

9. Leek and Potato Soup

Ingredients
- 2 tablespoons olive oil
- 3 leeks, cleaned and sliced
- 3 cloves garlic, minced
- 4 medium potatoes, peeled and diced
- 4 cups low-sodium vegetable broth
- 1 cup water
- 1 teaspoon dried thyme
- 1/2 cup low-fat milk
- Fresh chives for garnish

Instructions
1. Heat olive oil in a large pot over medium heat. Add leeks and garlic, and sauté until softened, about 5 minutes.
2. Add potatoes, vegetable broth, water, and thyme. Bring to a boil.
3. Reduce heat and simmer for 25-30 minutes, or until the potatoes are tender.
4. Use an immersion blender to puree the soup until smooth.
5. Stir in low-fat milk and heat through.
6. Serve hot, garnished with fresh chives.

Nutrition Info per Serving
- Calories: 200
- Protein: 4g
- Carbohydrates: 33g
- Dietary Fiber: 5g
- Sugars: 4g
- Fat: 7g
- Saturated Fat: 1g
- Sodium: 120mg

Serves
4 servings
Cooking Time
35 minutes

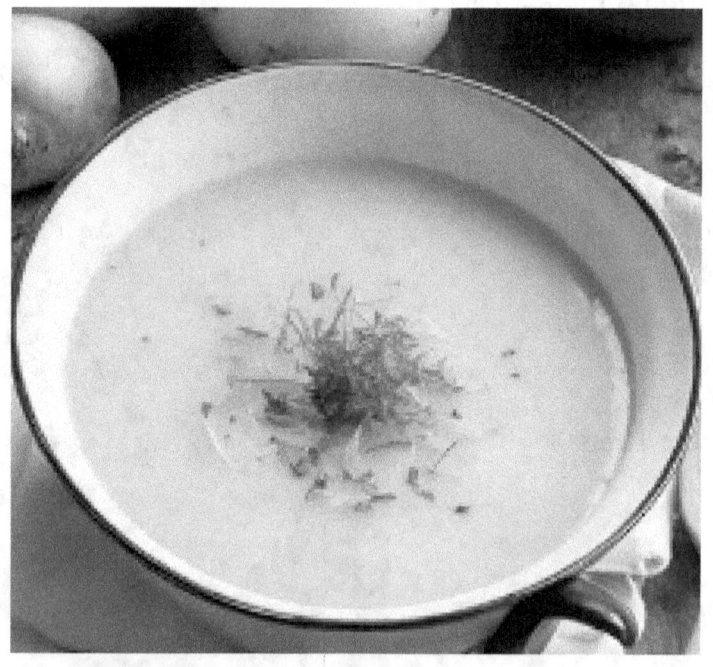

10. Cauliflower Soup

Ingredients
- 2 tablespoons olive oil
- 1 large onion, diced
- 3 cloves garlic, minced
- 1 large head of cauliflower, cut into florets
- 4 cups low-sodium vegetable broth
- 1 cup low-fat milk
- 1 teaspoon dried thyme
- 1 teaspoon ground cumin
- Fresh chives for garnish

Instructions
1. Heat olive oil in a large pot over medium heat. Add onion and garlic, and sauté until softened, about 5 minutes.
2. Add cauliflower florets, vegetable broth, thyme, and cumin. Bring to a boil.
3. Reduce heat and simmer for 20-25 minutes, or until the cauliflower is tender.
4. Use an immersion blender to puree the soup until smooth.
5. Stir in low-fat milk and heat through.
6. Serve hot, garnished with fresh chives.

Nutrition Info per Serving
- Calories: 150
- Protein: 4g
- Carbohydrates: 18g
- Dietary Fiber: 5g
- Sugars: 6g
- Fat: 7g
- Saturated Fat: 1.5g
- Sodium: 110mg

Serves
4 servings
Cooking Time
30 minutes

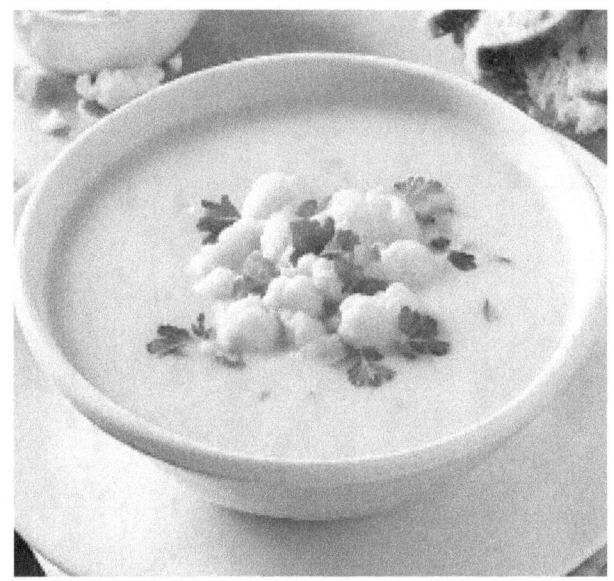

11. Cabbage Soup

Ingredients
- 2 tablespoons olive oil
- 1 large onion, diced
- 3 cloves garlic, minced
- 4 cups green cabbage, shredded
- 2 carrots, diced
- 2 celery stalks, diced
- 4 cups low-sodium vegetable broth
- 1 can (15 ounces) no-salt-added diced tomatoes
- 1 teaspoon dried thyme
- 1 teaspoon dried basil
- Fresh parsley for garnish

Instructions
1. Heat olive oil in a large pot over medium heat. Add onion and garlic, and sauté until softened, about 5 minutes.
2. Add cabbage, carrots, and celery, and cook for another 5 minutes.
3. Stir in vegetable broth, diced tomatoes, thyme, and basil. Bring to a boil.
4. Reduce heat and simmer for 30-35 minutes, or until the vegetables are tender.
5. Serve hot, garnished with fresh parsley.

Nutrition Info per Serving
- Calories: 130
- Protein: 3g
- Carbohydrates: 20g
- Dietary Fiber: 6g
- Sugars: 10g
- Fat: 5g
- Saturated Fat: 1g
- Sodium: 110mg

Serves
6 servings

Cooking Time
40 minutes

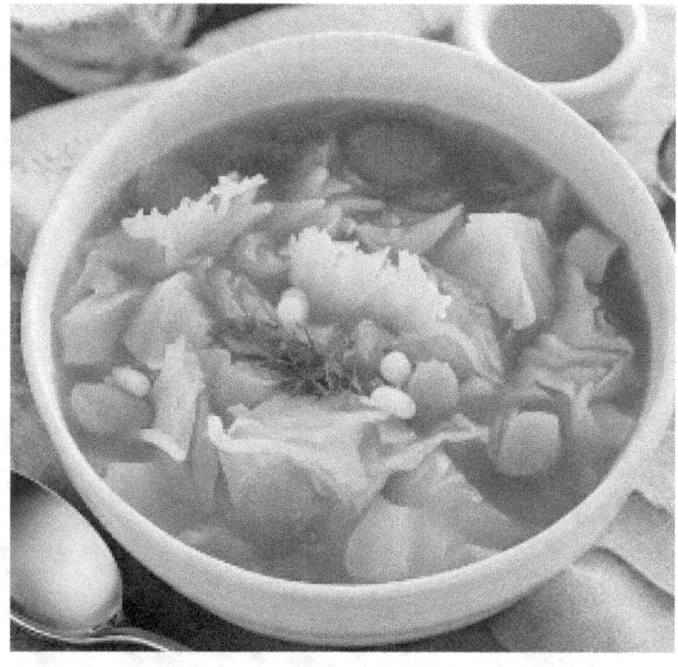

12. Sweet Potato and Apple Soup

Ingredients
- 2 tablespoons olive oil
- 1 large onion, diced
- 3 cloves garlic, minced
- 2 large sweet potatoes, peeled and diced
- 2 large apples, peeled, cored, and diced
- 4 cups low-sodium vegetable broth
- 1 teaspoon ground cinnamon
- 1/2 teaspoon ground nutmeg
- 1/2 teaspoon ground ginger
- Fresh thyme for garnish

Instructions
1. Heat olive oil in a large pot over medium heat. Add onion and garlic, and sauté until softened, about 5 minutes.
2. Add sweet potatoes, apples, vegetable broth, cinnamon, nutmeg, and ginger. Bring to a boil.
3. Reduce heat and simmer for 20-25 minutes, or until the sweet potatoes and apples are tender.
4. Use an immersion blender to puree the soup until smooth.
5. Serve hot, garnished with fresh thyme.

Nutrition Info per Serving
- Calories: 180
- Protein: 2g
- Carbohydrates: 32g
- Dietary Fiber: 5g
- Sugars: 15g
- Fat: 6g
- Saturated Fat: 1g
- Sodium: 100mg

Serves
4 servings
Cooking Time
30 minutes

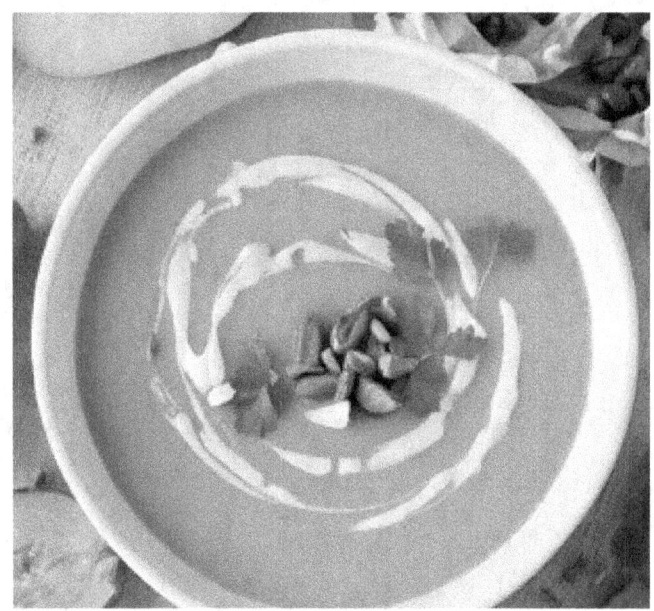

13. Asian Vegetable Soup

Ingredients
- 2 tablespoons sesame oil
- 1 large onion, diced
- 3 cloves garlic, minced
- 1 tablespoon fresh ginger, grated
- 4 cups low-sodium vegetable broth
- 1 cup water
- 1 cup sliced mushrooms
- 1 cup sliced carrots
- 1 cup snow peas
- 1 cup baby bok choy, chopped
- 1 tablespoon low-sodium soy sauce
- 1 teaspoon rice vinegar
- Fresh cilantro for garnish

Instructions
1. Heat sesame oil in a large pot over medium heat. Add onion, garlic, and ginger, and sauté until softened, about 5 minutes.
2. Add vegetable broth, water, mushrooms, carrots, snow peas, and bok choy. Bring to a boil.
3. Reduce heat and simmer for 15-20 minutes, or until the vegetables are tender.
4. Stir in soy sauce and rice vinegar.
5. Serve hot, garnished with fresh cilantro.

Nutrition Info per Serving
- Calories: 140
- Protein: 3g
- Carbohydrates: 15g
- Dietary Fiber: 5g
- Sugars: 7g
- Fat: 7g
- Saturated Fat: 1g
- Sodium: 120mg

Serves
4 servings
Cooking Time
25 minutes

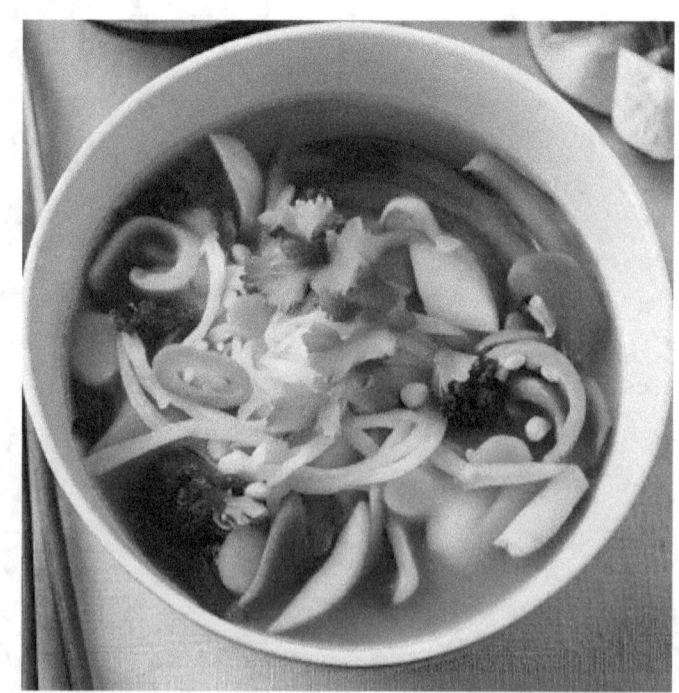

14. Broccoli and Stilton Soup

Ingredients
- 2 tablespoons olive oil
- 1 large onion, diced
- 3 cloves garlic, minced
- 4 cups broccoli florets
- 4 cups low-sodium vegetable broth
- 1 cup low-fat milk
- 1/4 cup crumbled Stilton cheese (low sodium)
- 1 teaspoon dried thyme
- Fresh chives for garnish

Instructions
1. Heat olive oil in a large pot over medium heat. Add onion and garlic, and sauté until softened, about 5 minutes.
2. Add broccoli, vegetable broth, and thyme. Bring to a boil.
3. Reduce heat and simmer for 20-25 minutes, or until the broccoli is tender.
4. Use an immersion blender to puree the soup until smooth.
5. Stir in low-fat milk and Stilton cheese, and heat through until the cheese is melted.
6. Serve hot, garnished with fresh chives.

Nutrition Info per Serving
- Calories: 170
- Protein: 7g
- Carbohydrates: 15g
- Dietary Fiber: 5g
- Sugars: 5g
- Fat: 9g
- Saturated Fat: 3g
- Sodium: 130mg

Serves
4 servings

Cooking Time
30 minutes

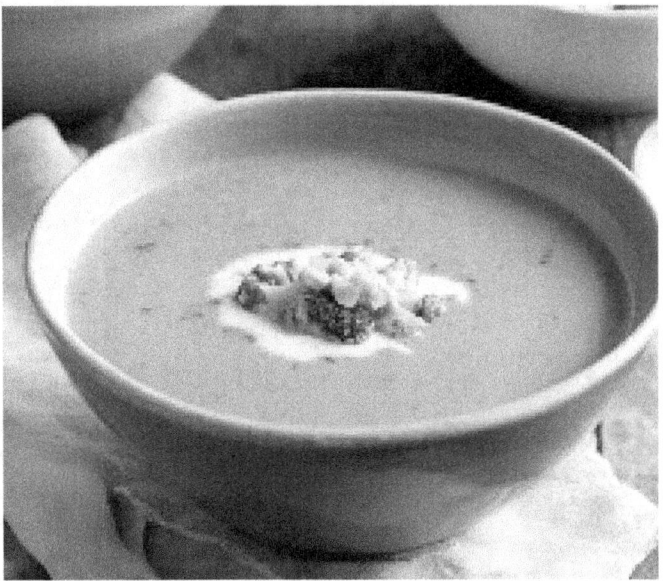

15. Panzanella Salad

Ingredients

- 4 cups stale whole wheat bread, cut into cubes
- 2 large tomatoes, diced
- 1 cucumber, peeled and diced
- 1 red bell pepper, diced
- 1 small red onion, thinly sliced
- 1/4 cup fresh basil leaves, chopped
- 3 tablespoons olive oil
- 2 tablespoons red wine vinegar
- 1 teaspoon dried oregano
- Fresh ground black pepper (optional)

Instructions

1. Preheat the oven to 350°F (175°C).
2. Spread the bread cubes on a baking sheet and bake for 10-12 minutes until lightly toasted. Let cool.
3. In a large bowl, combine tomatoes, cucumber, bell pepper, red onion, and basil.
4. Add the cooled bread cubes to the bowl.
5. In a small bowl, whisk together olive oil, red wine vinegar, and oregano.
6. Drizzle the dressing over the salad and toss to combine.
7. Let the salad sit for 10-15 minutes to allow the flavors to meld.
8. Serve immediately.

Nutrition Info per Serving

- Calories: 220
- Protein: 5g
- Carbohydrates: 28g
- Dietary Fiber: 5g
- Sugars: 7g
- Fat: 11g
- Saturated Fat: 1.5g
- Sodium: 80mg

Serves
4 servings
Cooking Time
25 minutes

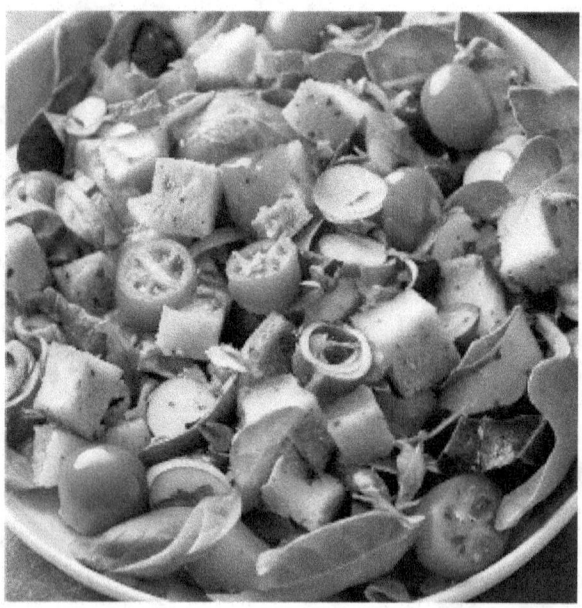

16. Endive and Orange Salad

Ingredients

- 4 endives, thinly sliced
- 2 large oranges, peeled and segmented
- 1/4 cup walnuts, chopped (unsalted)
- 1/4 cup crumbled goat cheese (low sodium)
- 2 tablespoons olive oil
- 1 tablespoon fresh lemon juice
- 1 teaspoon honey
- 1 teaspoon Dijon mustard (low sodium)

Instructions

1. In a large bowl, combine endives, orange segments, walnuts, and goat cheese.
2. In a small bowl, whisk together olive oil, lemon juice, honey, and Dijon mustard.
3. Drizzle the dressing over the salad and toss to combine.
4. Serve immediately.

Nutrition Info per Serving

- Calories: 180
- Protein: 4g
- Carbohydrates: 17g
- Dietary Fiber: 6g
- Sugars: 12g
- Fat: 11g
- Saturated Fat: 3g
- Sodium: 75mg

Serves
4 servings
Cooking Time
10 minutes

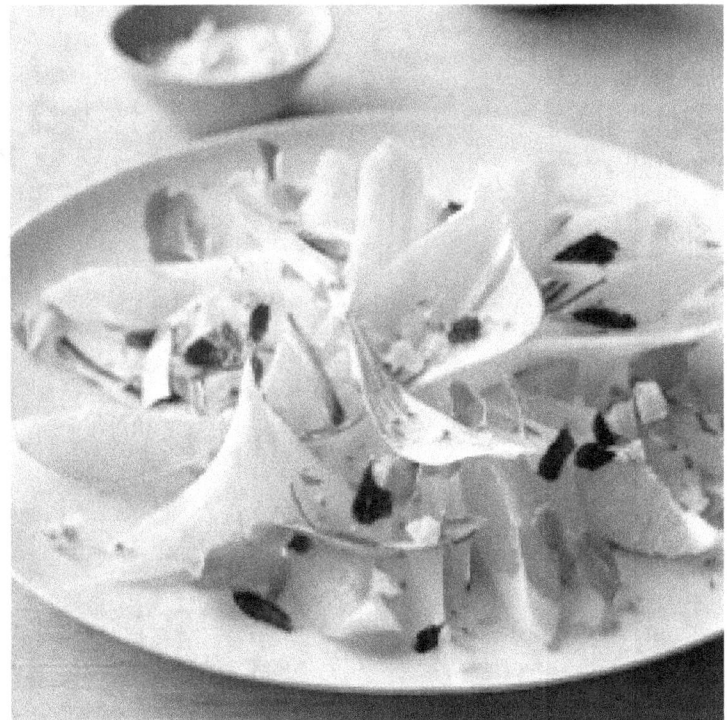

17. Summer Corn Salad

Ingredients

- 4 ears of corn, kernels removed
- 1 cup cherry tomatoes, halved
- 1 cucumber, diced
- 1 red bell pepper, diced
- 1/4 cup red onion, finely chopped
- 1/4 cup fresh basil leaves, chopped
- 3 tablespoons olive oil
- 2 tablespoons apple cider vinegar
- 1 teaspoon honey
- Fresh ground black pepper (optional)

Instructions

1. In a large bowl, combine corn kernels, cherry tomatoes, cucumber, red bell pepper, red onion, and basil.
2. In a small bowl, whisk together olive oil, apple cider vinegar, and honey.
3. Drizzle the dressing over the salad and toss to combine.
4. Serve immediately.

Nutrition Info per Serving

- Calories: 180
- Protein: 3g
- Carbohydrates: 24g
- Dietary Fiber: 4g
- Sugars: 8g
- Fat: 10g
- Saturated Fat: 1.5g
- Sodium: 20mg

Serves

4 servings

Cooking Time

15 minutes

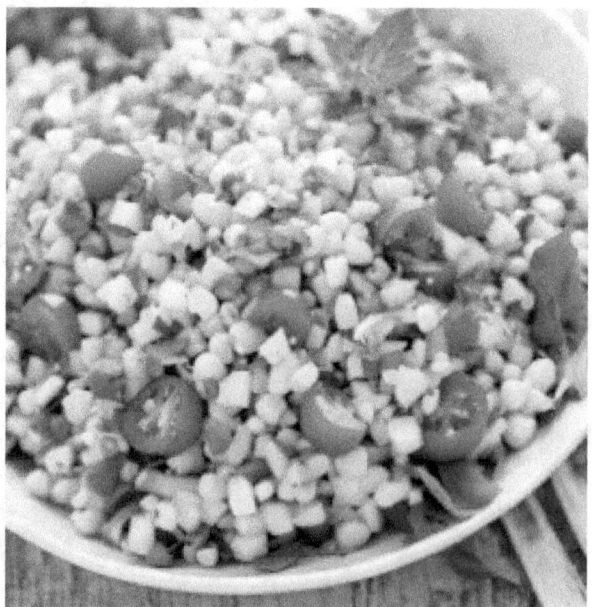

18. Mediterranean Chickpea Salad

Ingredients
- 1 can (15 ounces) no-salt-added chickpeas, drained and rinsed
- 1 cup cherry tomatoes, halved
- 1 cucumber, diced
- 1/4 cup red onion, finely chopped
- 1/4 cup Kalamata olives, pitted and sliced (low sodium)
- 1/4 cup feta cheese, crumbled (low sodium)
- 2 tablespoons fresh parsley, chopped
- 3 tablespoons olive oil
- 2 tablespoons lemon juice
- 1 teaspoon dried oregano
- Fresh ground black pepper (optional)

Instructions
1. In a large bowl, combine chickpeas, cherry tomatoes, cucumber, red onion, olives, feta cheese, and parsley.
2. In a small bowl, whisk together olive oil, lemon juice, and oregano.
3. Drizzle the dressing over the salad and toss to combine.
4. Serve immediately.

Nutrition Info per Serving
- Calories: 220
- Protein: 6g
- Carbohydrates: 20g
- Dietary Fiber: 5g
- Sugars: 4g
- Fat: 14g
- Saturated Fat: 3g
- Sodium: 140mg

Serves
4 servings

Cooking Time
10 minutes

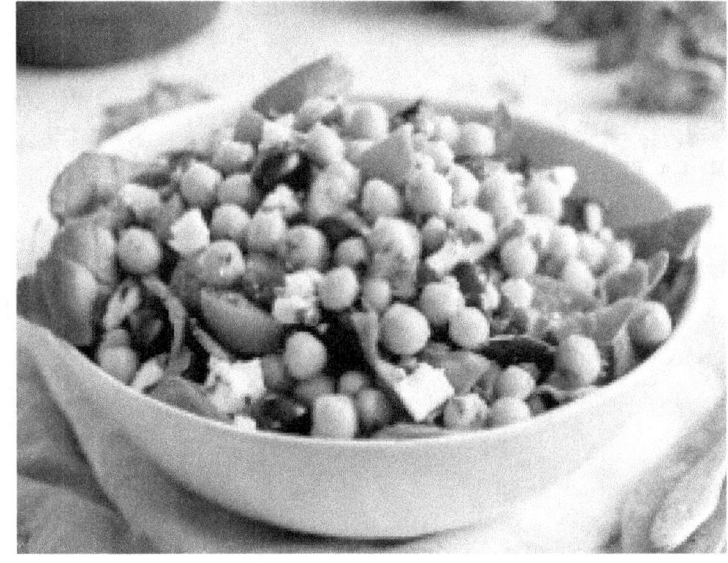

19. Waldorf Salad

Ingredients
- 2 large apples, cored and diced
- 1 cup red grapes, halved
- 1 cup celery, diced
- 1/2 cup walnuts, chopped (unsalted)
- 1/4 cup plain Greek yogurt (low-fat)
- 2 tablespoons mayonnaise (low sodium)
- 1 tablespoon lemon juice
- 1 teaspoon honey

Instructions
1. In a large bowl, combine apples, grapes, celery, and walnuts.
2. In a small bowl, whisk together Greek yogurt, mayonnaise, lemon juice, and honey.
3. Pour the dressing over the salad and toss to combine.
4. Serve immediately.

Nutrition Info per Serving
- Calories: 180
- Protein: 3g
- Carbohydrates: 22g
- Dietary Fiber: 4g
- Sugars: 15g
- Fat: 9g
- Saturated Fat: 1g
- Sodium: 40mg

Serves
4 servings

Cooking Time
10 minutes

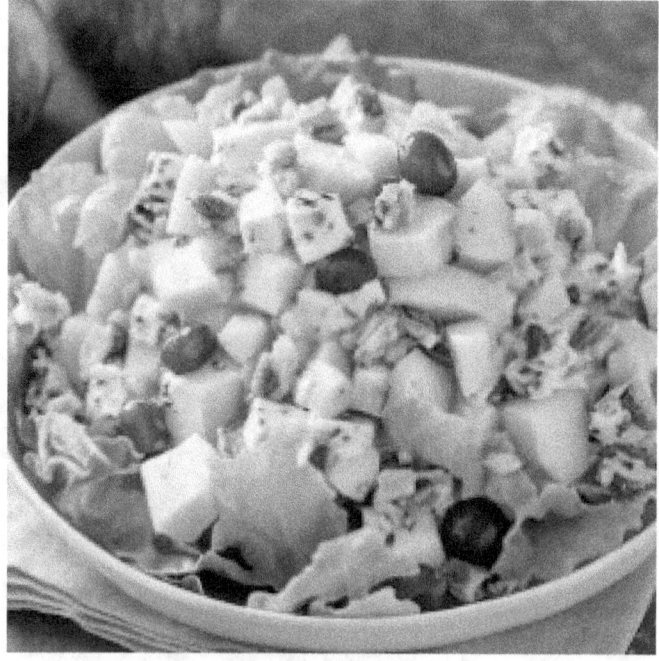

20. Asian Slaw

Ingredients

- 4 cups shredded cabbage
- 1 cup shredded carrots
- 1 red bell pepper, thinly sliced
- 1/4 cup green onions, thinly sliced
- 1/4 cup fresh cilantro, chopped
- 3 tablespoons rice vinegar
- 2 tablespoons olive oil
- 1 tablespoon low-sodium soy sauce
- 1 teaspoon honey
- 1 teaspoon sesame oil
- Fresh ground black pepper (optional)

Instructions

1. In a large bowl, combine cabbage, carrots, red bell pepper, green onions, and cilantro.
2. In a small bowl, whisk together rice vinegar, olive oil, soy sauce, honey, and sesame oil.
3. Pour the dressing over the slaw and toss to combine.
4. Serve immediately.

Nutrition Info per Serving

- Calories: 120
- Protein: 2g
- Carbohydrates: 12g
- Dietary Fiber: 4g
- Sugars: 7g
- Fat: 8g
- Saturated Fat: 1g
- Sodium: 80mg

Serves
4 servings
Cooking Time
10 minutes

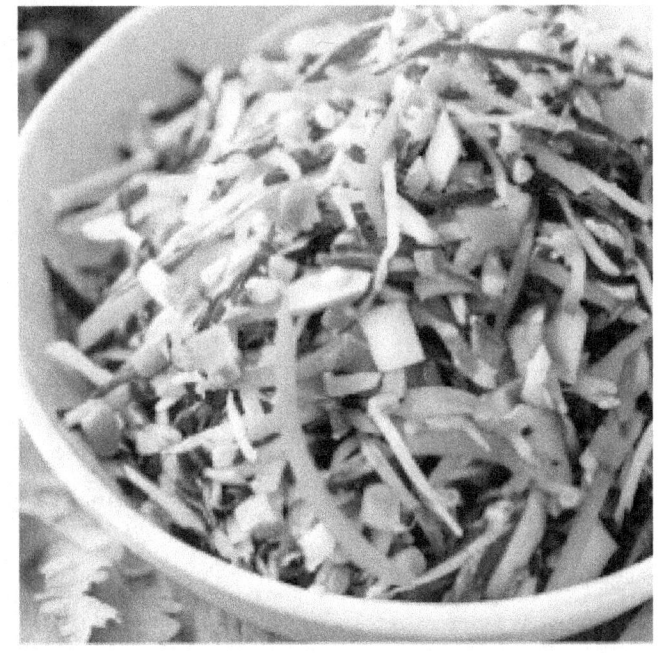

21. Spinach and Strawberry Salad

Ingredients
- 6 cups baby spinach leaves
- 1 cup strawberries, sliced
- 1/4 cup red onion, thinly sliced
- 1/4 cup walnuts, chopped (unsalted)
- 1/4 cup crumbled feta cheese (low sodium)
- 3 tablespoons olive oil
- 2 tablespoons balsamic vinegar
- 1 teaspoon honey
- Fresh ground black pepper (optional)

Instructions
1. In a large bowl, combine spinach, strawberries, red onion, walnuts, and feta cheese.
2. In a small bowl, whisk together olive oil, balsamic vinegar, and honey.
3. Drizzle the dressing over the salad and toss to combine.
4. Serve immediately.

Nutrition Info per Serving
- Calories: 170
- Protein: 4g
- Carbohydrates: 12g
- Dietary Fiber: 4g
- Sugars: 8g
- Fat: 13g
- Saturated Fat: 3g
- Sodium: 80mg

Serves
4 servings
Cooking Time
10 minutes

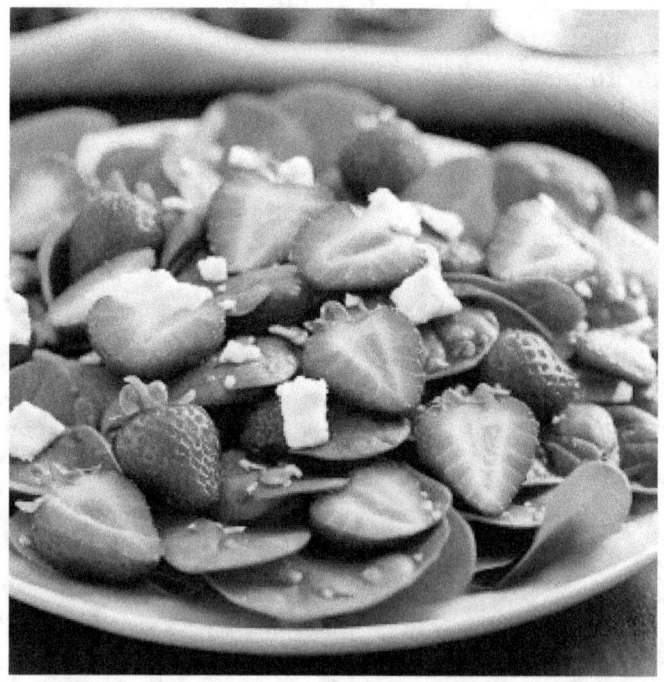

Snacks & Desserts

1. Tiramisu
Ingredients
- 1 cup brewed coffee, cooled
- 2 tablespoons coffee liqueur (optional)
- 24 ladyfingers (low sodium)
- 8 ounces mascarpone cheese (low sodium)
- 1 cup heavy cream
- 1/4 cup granulated sugar
- 1 teaspoon vanilla extract
- 2 tablespoons unsweetened cocoa powder
- Dark chocolate shavings for garnish (optional)

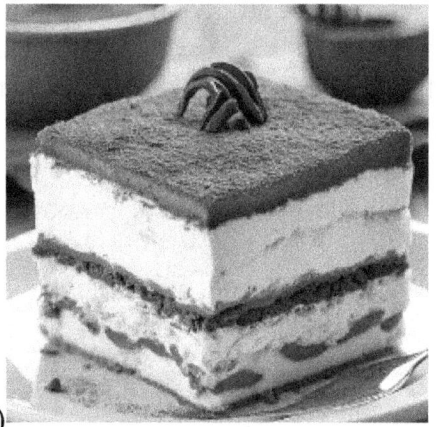

Instructions
1. In a shallow dish, combine the brewed coffee and coffee liqueur (if using).
2. Dip each ladyfinger briefly in the coffee mixture and arrange them in a single layer in an 8x8-inch dish.
3. In a large bowl, whisk the mascarpone cheese until smooth.
4. In another bowl, whip the heavy cream with the granulated sugar and vanilla extract until stiff peaks form.
5. Gently fold the whipped cream into the mascarpone cheese until well combined.
6. Spread half of the mascarpone mixture over the ladyfingers in the dish.
7. Add another layer of coffee-dipped ladyfingers on top of the mascarpone mixture.
8. Spread the remaining mascarpone mixture over the second layer of ladyfingers.
9. Dust the top with unsweetened cocoa powder.
10. Refrigerate for at least 4 hours or overnight.
11. Garnish with dark chocolate shavings before serving, if desired.

Nutrition Info per Serving
- Calories: 250 Protein: 4g Carbohydrates: 24g   Dietary Fiber: 1g
- Sugars: 10g
- Fat: 15g
- Saturated Fat: 9g
- Sodium: 70mg

Serves
8 servings
Cooking Time
15 minutes (plus chilling time)

2. Chocolate Covered Strawberries

Ingredients
- 1 pound fresh strawberries, washed and dried
- 8 ounces dark chocolate (70% cocoa), chopped
- 1 tablespoon coconut oil

Instructions
1. Line a baking sheet with parchment paper.
2. In a microwave-safe bowl, combine the dark chocolate and coconut oil.
3. Microwave in 30-second intervals, stirring between each interval, until the chocolate is melted and smooth.
4. Dip each strawberry into the melted chocolate, allowing the excess to drip off.
5. Place the dipped strawberries on the prepared baking sheet.
6. Refrigerate for at least 30 minutes until the chocolate is set.
7. Serve chilled.

Nutrition Info per Serving
- Calories: 100
- Protein: 1g
- Carbohydrates: 12g
- Dietary Fiber: 2g
- Sugars: 9g
- Fat: 6g
- Saturated Fat: 4g
- Sodium: 5mg

Serves

12 servings

Cooking Time

10 minutes (plus chilling time)

3. Mango Lassi

Ingredients
- 2 ripe mangoes, peeled and diced
- 1 cup plain Greek yogurt (low-fat)
- 1/2 cup unsweetened almond milk
- 1 tablespoon honey
- 1/2 teaspoon ground cardamom
- Ice cubes (optional)

Instructions
1. In a blender, combine the diced mangoes, Greek yogurt, almond milk, honey, and ground cardamom.
2. Blend until smooth.
3. Add ice cubes if desired and blend again.
4. Pour into glasses and serve immediately.

Nutrition Info per Serving
- Calories: 150
- Protein: 6g
- Carbohydrates: 30g
- Dietary Fiber: 2g
- Sugars: 25g
- Fat: 2g
- Saturated Fat: 1g
- Sodium: 60mg

Serves
2 servings
Cooking Time
5 minutes

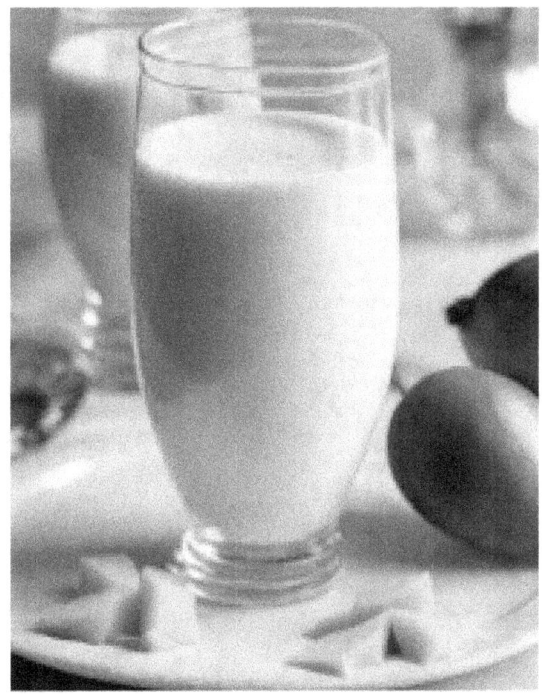

4. Orange Gelatin

Ingredients
- 1 cup freshly squeezed orange juice
- 1 tablespoon unflavored gelatin
- 2 tablespoons honey
- 1 cup water
- Orange segments for garnish (optional)
- Fresh mint leaves for garnish (optional)

Instructions
1. In a small saucepan, combine water and honey. Heat over medium heat until the honey is dissolved.
2. Remove from heat and sprinkle the gelatin over the mixture. Let it sit for 1 minute to bloom.
3. Stir in the freshly squeezed orange juice until the gelatin is completely dissolved.
4. Pour the mixture into serving glasses or a mold.
5. Refrigerate for at least 4 hours until set.
6. Garnish with orange segments and fresh mint leaves before serving, if desired.

Nutrition Info per Serving
- Calories: 60
- Protein: 1g
- Carbohydrates: 15g
- Dietary Fiber: 0g
- Sugars: 13g
- Fat: 0g
- Saturated Fat: 0g
- Sodium: 5mg

Serves
4 servings

Cooking Time
10 minutes (plus chilling time)

5. Strawberry Shortcake

Ingredients
- Shortcakes:
    - 2 cups whole wheat flour
    - 2 tablespoons granulated sugar
    - 1 tablespoon baking powder (low sodium)
    - 1/2 cup unsalted butter, cold and cut into cubes
    - 2/3 cup low-fat milk
- Strawberries:
    - 4 cups fresh strawberries, hulled and sliced
    - 2 tablespoons honey
- Whipped Cream:
    - 1 cup heavy cream
    - 1 tablespoon honey
    - 1 teaspoon vanilla extract

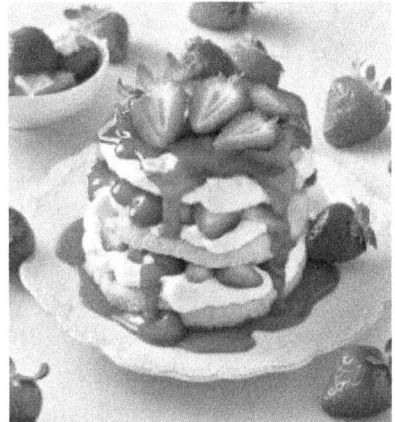

Instructions
1. **For the Shortcakes:**
    a. Preheat the oven to 400°F (200°C).
    b. In a large bowl, combine the flour, sugar, and baking powder.
    c. Cut in the butter until the mixture resembles coarse crumbs.
    d. Stir in the milk until just combined.
    e. Drop the dough by spoonfuls onto a baking sheet lined with parchment paper.
    f. Bake for 15-18 minutes or until golden brown. Let cool.
2. **For the Strawberries:**
    a. In a medium bowl, mix the sliced strawberries with honey. Let sit for at least 10 minutes to macerate.
3. **For the Whipped Cream:**
    a. In a large bowl, whip the heavy cream with honey and vanilla extract until stiff peaks form.
4. To Assemble:
    a. Split the shortcakes in half and layer with strawberries and whipped cream.
    b. Serve immediately.

Nutrition Info per Serving
- Calories: 250   Protein: 4g   Carbohydrates: 28g   Dietary Fiber: 4g
- Sugars: 12g   Fat: 14g   Saturated Fat: 8g
- Sodium: 60mg

Serves

8 servings

Cooking Time

30 minutes

6. Fig Bars

Ingredients
- **Crust and Topping:**
    - 1 1/2 cups rolled oats
    - 1 cup whole wheat flour
    - 1/2 cup unsalted butter, melted
    - 1/4 cup honey
- **Fig Filling:**
    - 1 cup dried figs, chopped
    - 1/2 cup water
    - 2 tablespoons honey
    - 1 teaspoon vanilla extract

Instructions
1. **For the Fig Filling:**
    a. In a small saucepan, combine figs, water, and honey. Bring to a boil, then reduce heat and simmer for 10 minutes until the figs are soft.
    b. Remove from heat and stir in vanilla extract. Puree the mixture in a food processor until smooth.
2. **For the Crust and Topping:**
    a. Preheat the oven to 350°F (175°C).
    b. In a large bowl, mix oats, flour, melted butter, and honey until crumbly.
    c. Press half of the mixture into a greased 8x8-inch baking pan.
    d. Spread the fig filling evenly over the crust.
    e. Sprinkle the remaining oat mixture over the fig filling, pressing gently.
    f. Bake for 25-30 minutes or until golden brown. Let cool completely before cutting into bars.

Nutrition Info per Serving
- Calories: 180
- Protein: 3g
- Carbohydrates: 27g
- Dietary Fiber: 3g
- Sugars: 15g
- Fat: 7g
- Saturated Fat: 4g
- Sodium: 20mg

Serves
12 servings
Cooking Time
40 minutes

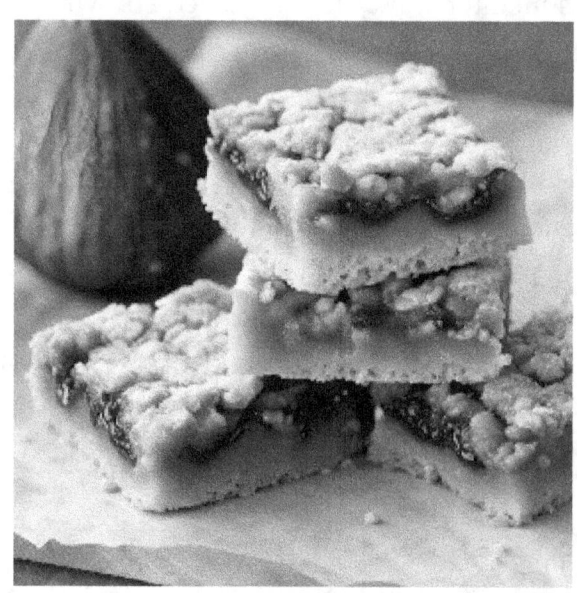

7. Almond Joy Bites

Ingredients
- 1 cup unsweetened shredded coconut
- 1/4 cup honey
- 1/4 cup coconut oil, melted
- 1/2 teaspoon vanilla extract
- 24 whole almonds
- 4 ounces dark chocolate (70% cocoa), melted

Instructions
1. In a medium bowl, combine shredded coconut, honey, coconut oil, and vanilla extract until well mixed.
2. Form the mixture into small balls, placing an almond in the center of each.
3. Place the balls on a baking sheet lined with parchment paper and freeze for 15 minutes.
4. Dip each ball into the melted dark chocolate, allowing the excess to drip off.
5. Place the chocolate-covered bites back on the parchment paper and refrigerate until the chocolate is set.
6. Serve chilled.

Nutrition Info per Serving
- Calories: 90
- Protein: 1g
- Carbohydrates: 8g
- Dietary Fiber: 2g
- Sugars: 6g
- Fat: 7g
- Saturated Fat: 5g
- Sodium: 5mg

Serves
24 bites

Cooking Time
30 minutes (plus chilling time)

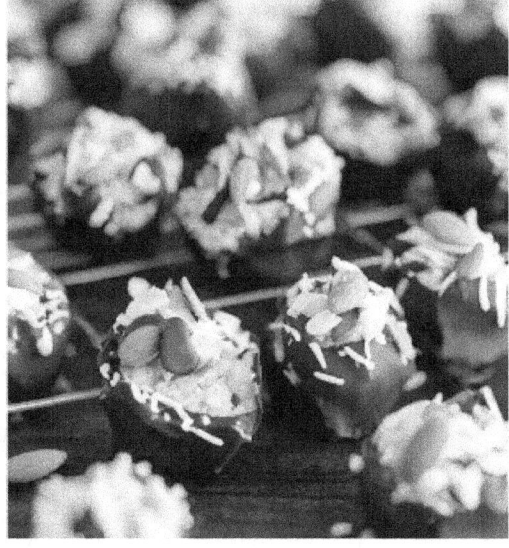

8. Banana Bread

Ingredients
- 3 ripe bananas, mashed
- 1/3 cup melted coconut oil
- 1/4 cup honey
- 1 large egg
- 1 teaspoon vanilla extract
- 1 teaspoon baking soda (low sodium)
- 1/4 teaspoon ground cinnamon
- 1 1/2 cups whole wheat flour

Instructions
1. Preheat the oven to 350°F (175°C). Grease a 9x5-inch loaf pan.
2. In a large bowl, combine mashed bananas, melted coconut oil, honey, egg, and vanilla extract.
3. Stir in baking soda and cinnamon.
4. Add the whole wheat flour and mix until just combined.
5. Pour the batter into the prepared loaf pan.
6. Bake for 50-60 minutes, or until a toothpick inserted into the center comes out clean.
7. Let cool in the pan for 10 minutes before transferring to a wire rack to cool completely.
8. Slice and serve.

Nutrition Info per Serving
- Calories: 180
- Protein: 3g
- Carbohydrates: 30g
- Dietary Fiber: 3g
- Sugars: 12g
- Fat: 6g
- Saturated Fat: 4g
- Sodium: 80mg

Serves
12 slices

Cooking Time
60 minutes

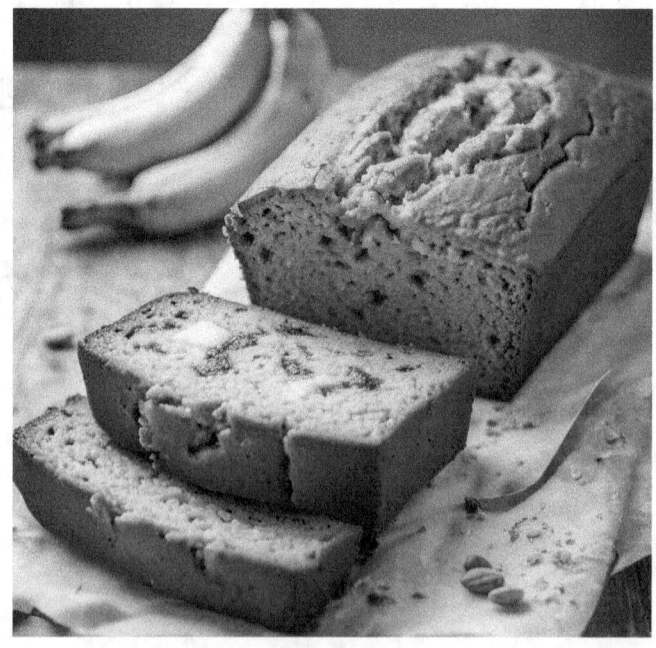

9. Pumpkin Pie

Ingredients
- **Crust:**
  - 1 1/2 cups whole wheat flour
  - 1/2 cup cold unsalted butter, cubed
  - 2-4 tablespoons cold water
- **Filling:**
  - 1 can (15 ounces) pumpkin puree (no added salt)
  - 1/2 cup honey
  - 2 large eggs
  - 1 cup low-fat milk
  - 1 teaspoon ground cinnamon
  - 1/2 teaspoon ground ginger
  - 1/4 teaspoon ground nutmeg
  - 1/4 teaspoon ground cloves

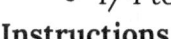

Instructions
1. **For the Crust:**
   a. In a food processor, combine whole wheat flour and cold butter. Pulse until the mixture resembles coarse crumbs.
   b. Gradually add cold water, 1 tablespoon at a time, until the dough comes together.
   c. Roll the dough into a ball, wrap in plastic wrap, and refrigerate for 30 minutes.
   d. Preheat the oven to 375°F (190°C).
   e. Roll out the dough on a lightly floured surface and fit it into a 9-inch pie dish. Trim the edges and set aside.
2. **For the Filling:**
   a. In a large bowl, combine pumpkin puree, honey, eggs, milk, cinnamon, ginger, nutmeg, and cloves. Mix until smooth.
   b. Pour the filling into the prepared crust.
   c. Bake for 45-50 minutes, or until the filling is set and a toothpick inserted into the center comes out clean.
   d. Let the pie cool completely before serving.

Nutrition Info per Serving
- Calories: 220 Protein: 4g Carbohydrates: 30g Dietary Fiber: 4g
- Sugars: 15g Fat: 10g Saturated Fat: 6g Sodium: 60mg

Serves
8 servings

Cooking Time
60 minutes (plus chilling time)

10. Oatmeal Cookies

Ingredients
- 1 cup rolled oats
- 1/2 cup whole wheat flour
- 1/2 teaspoon baking soda (low sodium)
- 1/2 teaspoon ground cinnamon
- 1/4 cup unsalted butter, melted
- 1/4 cup honey
- 1 large egg
- 1 teaspoon vanilla extract
- 1/2 cup raisins

Instructions
1. Preheat the oven to 350°F (175°C). Line a baking sheet with parchment paper.
2. In a large bowl, combine rolled oats, whole wheat flour, baking soda, and cinnamon.
3. In another bowl, mix melted butter, honey, egg, and vanilla extract until well combined.
4. Add the wet ingredients to the dry ingredients and stir until combined.
5. Fold in the raisins.
6. Drop spoonfuls of dough onto the prepared baking sheet, spacing them about 2 inches apart.
7. Bake for 10-12 minutes, or until the edges are golden brown.
8. Let cool on the baking sheet for 5 minutes before transferring to a wire rack to cool completely.

Nutrition Info per Serving
- Calories: 90
- Protein: 2g
- Carbohydrates: 14g
- Dietary Fiber: 2g
- Sugars: 7g
- Fat: 3g
- Saturated Fat: 1.5g
- Sodium: 20mg

Serves
18 cookies

Cooking Time
15 minutes

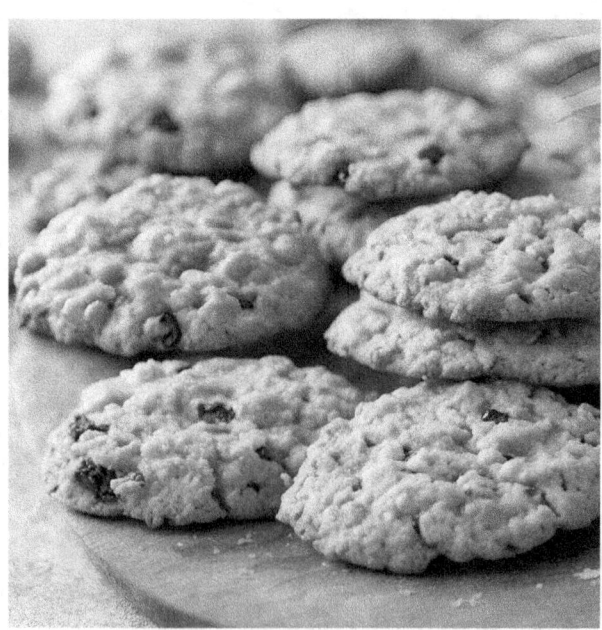

11. Cheese and Fruit Plate

Ingredients
- 1 cup grapes
- 1 apple, sliced
- 1 pear, sliced
- 1/2 cup strawberries, halved
- 4 ounces low-sodium cheese (such as Swiss or mozzarella), cubed
- 1/4 cup unsalted almonds

Instructions
1. Arrange the grapes, apple slices, pear slices, strawberries, cheese cubes, and almonds on a serving plate.
2. Serve immediately.

Nutrition Info per Serving
- Calories: 150
- Protein: 7g
- Carbohydrates: 18g
- Dietary Fiber: 4g
- Sugars: 14g
- Fat: 7g
- Saturated Fat: 3g
- Sodium: 80mg

Serves
4 servings
Cooking Time
5 minutes

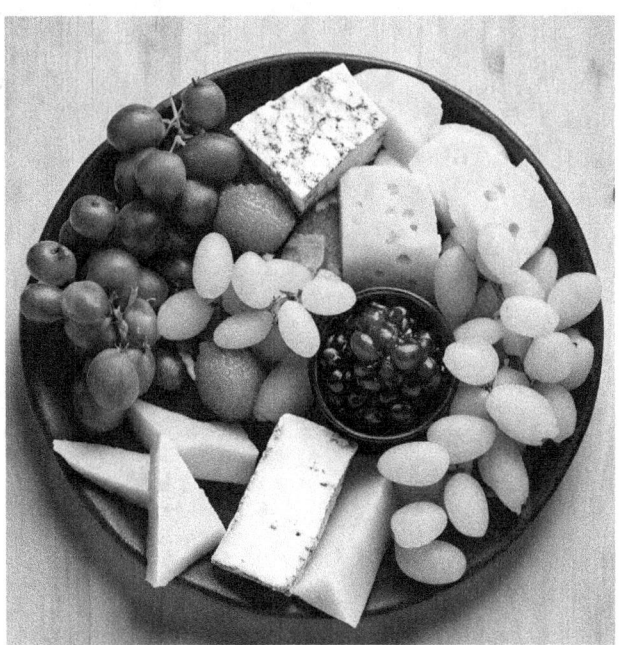

12. Baked Kale Chips

Ingredients
- 1 bunch kale, washed and dried
- 2 tablespoons olive oil
- 1 teaspoon garlic powder
- 1 teaspoon paprika

Instructions
1. Preheat the oven to 300°F (150°C). Line a baking sheet with parchment paper.
2. Remove the kale leaves from the stems and tear into bite-sized pieces.
3. In a large bowl, toss the kale with olive oil, garlic powder, and paprika.
4. Spread the kale evenly on the prepared baking sheet.
5. Bake for 20-25 minutes, or until the kale is crispy.
6. Let cool before serving.

Nutrition Info per Serving
- Calories: 50
- Protein: 2g
- Carbohydrates: 5g
- Dietary Fiber: 2g
- Sugars: 1g
- Fat: 3g
- Saturated Fat: 0.5g
- Sodium: 20mg

Serves
4 servings

Cooking Time
30 minutes

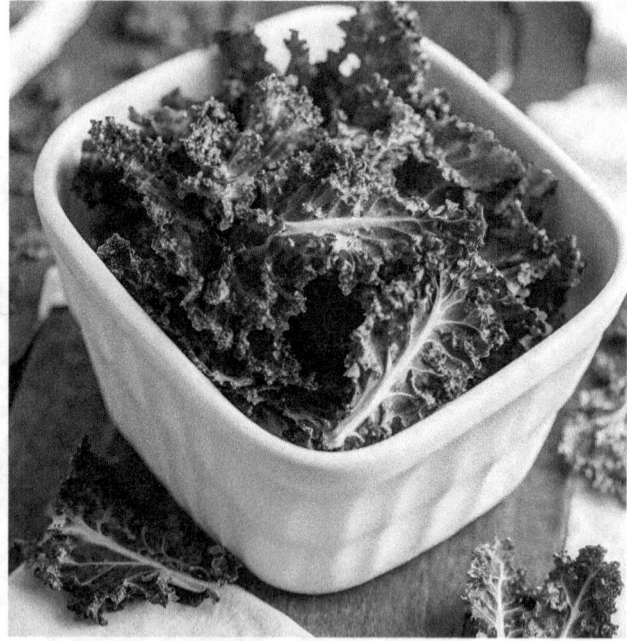

13. Frozen Yogurt Bark

Ingredients
- 2 cups plain Greek yogurt (low-fat)
- 2 tablespoons honey
- 1/2 cup mixed berries (such as blueberries, raspberries, and strawberries)
- 1/4 cup unsalted nuts, chopped

Instructions
1. Line a baking sheet with parchment paper.
2. In a bowl, mix the Greek yogurt and honey until well combined.
3. Spread the yogurt mixture evenly on the prepared baking sheet.
4. Sprinkle the mixed berries and chopped nuts over the yogurt.
5. Freeze for at least 3 hours, or until the yogurt is firm.
6. Break into pieces and serve.

Nutrition Info per Serving
- Calories: 100
- Protein: 8g
- Carbohydrates: 14g
- Dietary Fiber: 2g
- Sugars: 10g
- Fat: 3g
- Saturated Fat: 0.5g
- Sodium: 40mg

Serves
8 servings

Cooking Time
10 minutes (plus freezing time)

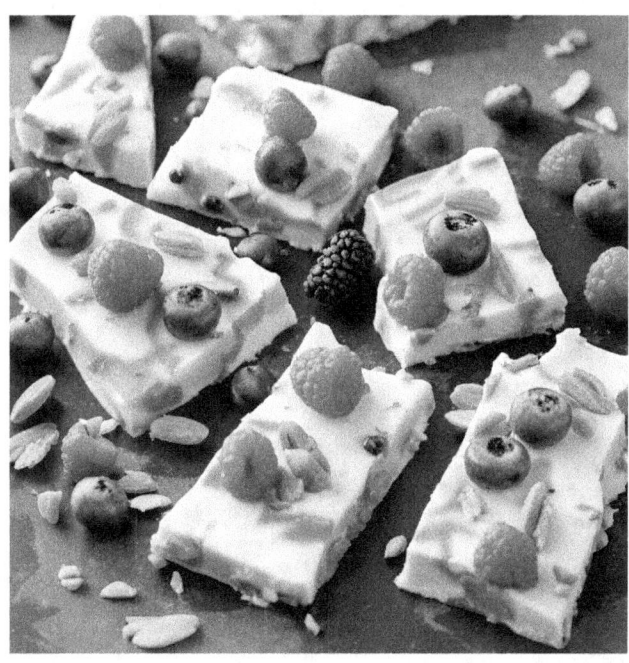

14. Cucumber Sandwiches

Ingredients
- 1 cucumber, thinly sliced
- 8 slices whole wheat bread
- 4 ounces low-sodium cream cheese
- 1 tablespoon fresh dill, chopped
- 1 teaspoon lemon juice

Instructions
1. In a small bowl, mix the cream cheese, dill, and lemon juice until well combined.
2. Spread the cream cheese mixture evenly on 4 slices of whole wheat bread.
3. Layer the cucumber slices on top of the cream cheese mixture.
4. Top with the remaining slices of bread.
5. Cut the sandwiches into quarters and serve.

Nutrition Info per Serving
- Calories: 120
- Protein: 5g
- Carbohydrates: 18g
- Dietary Fiber: 3g
- Sugars: 3g
- Fat: 4g
- Saturated Fat: 2g
- Sodium: 100mg

Serves
4 servings
Cooking Time
10 minutes

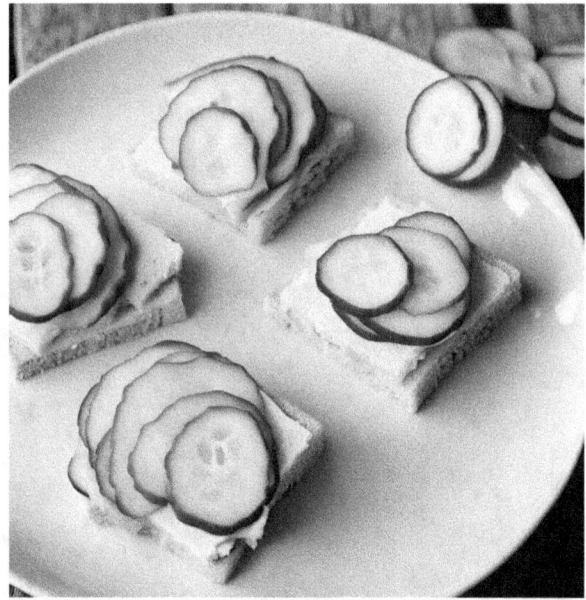

15. Vegetable Chips

Ingredients
- 1 sweet potato, thinly sliced
- 1 beet, thinly sliced
- 1 zucchini, thinly sliced
- 2 tablespoons olive oil
- 1 teaspoon paprika
- 1 teaspoon garlic powder

Instructions
1. Preheat the oven to 375°F (190°C). Line a baking sheet with parchment paper.
2. In a large bowl, toss the sweet potato, beet, and zucchini slices with olive oil, paprika, and garlic powder until well coated.
3. Arrange the vegetable slices in a single layer on the prepared baking sheet.
4. Bake for 20-25 minutes, flipping halfway through, until the chips are crispy.
5. Let cool before serving.

Nutrition Info per Serving
- Calories: 90
- Protein: 2g
- Carbohydrates: 14g
- Dietary Fiber: 3g
- Sugars: 5g
- Fat: 4g
- Saturated Fat: 0.5g
- Sodium: 15mg

Serves
4 servings
Cooking Time
30 minutes

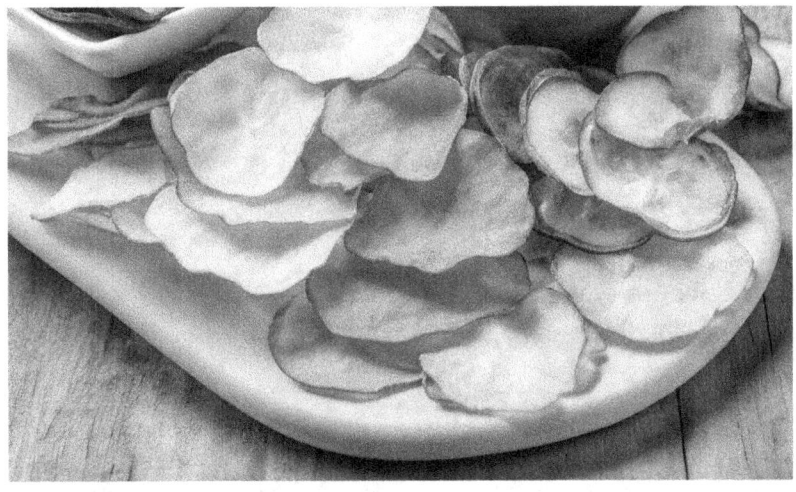

10-WEEK MEAL PLAN

Week 1

Monday
- Breakfast: Greek Yogurt with Nuts and Berries
- Lunch: Spinach and Strawberry Salad
- Dinner: Lemon Herb Baked Cod
- Snack: Almond Joy Bites

Tuesday
- Breakfast: Oatmeal Cookies
- Lunch: Beet and Goat Cheese Salad
- Dinner: Herb Roasted Chicken
- Snack: Cheese and Fruit Plate

Wednesday
- Breakfast: Pumpkin Spice Yogurt
- Lunch: Garden Vegetable Soup
- Dinner: Roasted Salmon with Dill
- Snack: Baked Kale Chips

Thursday
- Breakfast: Ricotta and Pear Toast
- Lunch: Endive and Orange Salad
- Dinner: Paprika Tilapia
- Snack: Frozen Yogurt Bark

Friday
- Breakfast: Cottage Cheese Pancakes
- Lunch: Mixed Greens with Apple Slices
- Dinner: Baked Haddock with Tomatoes
- Snack: Fig Bars

Saturday
- Breakfast: Almond Flour Pancakes
- Lunch: Mediterranean Chickpea Salad
- Dinner: Lemon Garlic Turkey Breast
- Snack: Cucumber Sandwiches

Sunday
- Breakfast: Buckwheat Pancakes
- Lunch: Summer Corn Salad
- Dinner: Chicken Piccata
- Snack: Vegetable Chips

Week 2

Monday
- Breakfast: Quinoa Porridge
- Lunch: Waldorf Salad
- Dinner: Barbecue Chicken
- Snack: Tiramisu

Tuesday
- Breakfast: Avocado Smoothie
- Lunch: Broccoli and Stilton Soup
- Dinner: Spiced Roast Turkey
- Snack: Chocolate Covered Strawberries

Wednesday
- Breakfast: Barley Porridge
- Lunch: Cabbage Soup
- Dinner: Grilled Swordfish with Salsa Verde
- Snack: Mango Lassi

Thursday
- Breakfast: Berry Banana Smoothie
- Lunch: Asian Vegetable Soup
- Dinner: Pesto Rubbed Chicken
- Snack: Orange Gelatin

Friday
- Breakfast: Pineapple Coconut Smoothie
- Lunch: Carrot and Coriander Soup
- Dinner: Mustard Roasted Trout
- Snack: Oatmeal Cookies

Saturday
- Breakfast: Sweet Potato Hash
- Lunch: Leek and Potato Soup
- Dinner: Turkey Burgers
- Snack: Cheese and Fruit Plate

Sunday
- Breakfast: Mushroom and Spinach Saute
- Lunch: Beetroot and Ginger Soup
- Dinner: Chili Lime Shrimp Skewers
- Snack: Baked Kale Chips

Week 3

Monday
- Breakfast: Frittata
- Lunch: Broccoli and Stilton Soup
- Dinner: Pan-Seared Scallops with Lemon
- Snack: Fig Bars

Tuesday
- Breakfast: Egg Muffins
- Lunch: Spinach and Strawberry Salad
- Dinner: Orange Glazed Halibut
- Snack: Frozen Yogurt Bark

Wednesday
- Breakfast: Pumpkin Spice Yogurt
- Lunch: Garden Vegetable Soup
- Dinner: Lemon Pepper Catfish
- Snack: Almond Joy Bites

Thursday
- Breakfast: Ricotta and Pear Toast
- Lunch: Endive and Orange Salad
- Dinner: Herbed Sea Bass
- Snack: Chocolate Covered Strawberries

Friday
- Breakfast: Cottage Cheese Pancakes
- Lunch: Mixed Greens with Apple Slices
- Dinner: Grilled Chicken with Chimichurri
- Snack: Tiramisu

Saturday
- Breakfast: Almond Flour Pancakes
- Lunch: Mediterranean Chickpea Salad
- Dinner: Turkey Scallopini
- Snack: Mango Lassi

Sunday
- Breakfast: Buckwheat Pancakes
- Lunch: Summer Corn Salad
- Dinner: Lemon Sole Meuniere
- Snack: Vegetable Chips

Week 4

Monday
- Breakfast: Quinoa Porridge
- Lunch: Waldorf Salad
- Dinner: Stir-Fried Turkey with Vegetables
- Snack: Orange Gelatin

Tuesday
- Breakfast: Avocado Smoothie
- Lunch: Cabbage Soup
- Dinner: Grilled Turkey Steaks
- Snack: Fig Bars

Wednesday
- Breakfast: Barley Porridge
- Lunch: Broccoli and Stilton Soup
- Dinner: Baked Scallops with Herbs
- Snack: Tiramisu

Thursday
- Breakfast: Berry Banana Smoothie
- Lunch: Asian Vegetable Soup
- Dinner: Pan-Seared Chicken with Spinach
- Snack: Baked Kale Chips

Friday
- Breakfast: Pineapple Coconut Smoothie
- Lunch: Carrot and Coriander Soup
- Dinner: Peppered Mackerel
- Snack: Chocolate Covered Strawberries

Saturday
- Breakfast: Sweet Potato Hash
- Lunch: Leek and Potato Soup
- Dinner: Tandoori Chicken
- Snack: Almond Joy Bites

Sunday
- Breakfast: Mushroom and Spinach Saute
- Lunch: Beetroot and Ginger Soup
- Dinner: Thai Grilled Chicken
- Snack: Frozen Yogurt Bark

Week 5

Monday
- Breakfast: Frittata
- Lunch: Spinach and Strawberry Salad
- Dinner: Grilled Sardines with Lemon
- Snack: Cheese and Fruit Plate

Tuesday
- Breakfast: Egg Muffins
- Lunch: Garden Vegetable Soup
- Dinner: Broiled Tilapia with Thyme
- Snack: Fig Bars

Wednesday
- Breakfast: Pumpkin Spice Yogurt
- Lunch: Mixed Greens with Apple Slices
- Dinner: Chicken Marsala
- Snack: Orange Gelatin

Thursday
- Breakfast: Ricotta and Pear Toast
- Lunch: Endive and Orange Salad
- Dinner: Mustard Roasted Trout
- Snack: Oatmeal Cookies

Friday
- Breakfast: Cottage Cheese Pancakes
- Lunch: Waldorf Salad
- Dinner: Orange Roast Chicken
- Snack: Chocolate Covered Strawberries

Saturday
- Breakfast: Almond Flour Pancakes
- Lunch: Mediterranean Chickpea Salad
- Dinner: Pan-Seared Scallops with Lemon
- Snack: Baked Kale Chips

Sunday
- Breakfast: Buckwheat Pancakes
- Lunch: Summer Corn Salad
- Dinner: Balsamic Glazed Chicken
- Snack: Frozen Yogurt Bark

Week 6

Monday
- Breakfast: Whole Wheat Toast
- Lunch: Split Pea Soup
- Dinner: Turkey and White Bean Chili
- Snack: Vegetable Chips

Tuesday
- Breakfast: Mango Lassi
- Lunch: Beetroot and Ginger Soup
- Dinner: Grilled Tuna with Basil Pesto
- Snack: Cheese and Fruit Plate

Wednesday
- Breakfast: Homemade Muesli Bread
- Lunch: Mixed Greens with Apple Slices
- Dinner: Lemon Chicken Orzo Soup
- Snack: Baked Kale Chips

Thursday
- Breakfast: Barley Porridge
- Lunch: Carrot and Coriander Soup
- Dinner: Sautéed Shrimp with Ginger and Honey
- Snack: Fig Bars

Friday
- Breakfast: Egg Muffins
- Lunch: Endive and Orange Salad
- Dinner: Pan-Seared Chicken with Spinach
- Snack: Tiramisu

Saturday
- Breakfast: Almond Flour Pancakes
- Lunch: Broccoli and Stilton Soup
- Dinner: Grilled Clams with Garlic
- Snack: Orange Gelatin

Sunday
- Breakfast: Pineapple Coconut Smoothie
- Lunch: Summer Corn Salad
- Dinner: Tom Yum Goong
- Snack: Almond Joy Bites

Week 7

Monday
- Breakfast: Sweet Potato Hash
- Lunch: Leek and Potato Soup
- Dinner: Mustard Roasted Trout
- Snack: Chocolate Covered Strawberries

Tuesday
- Breakfast: Quinoa Porridge
- Lunch: Spinach and Strawberry Salad
- Dinner: Pan-Seared Scallops with Lemon
- Snack: Baked Kale Chips

Wednesday
- Breakfast: Mushroom and Spinach Sauté
- Lunch: Cabbage Soup
- Dinner: Baked Haddock with Tomatoes
- Snack: Frozen Yogurt Bark

Thursday
- Breakfast: Buckwheat Porridge
- Lunch: Mediterranean Chickpea Salad
- Dinner: Lemon Sole Meuniere
- Snack: Cheese and Fruit Plate

Friday
- Breakfast: Egg Muffins
- Lunch: Waldorf Salad
- Dinner: Chicken Marsala
- Snack: Vegetable Chips

Saturday
- Breakfast: Cottage Cheese Pancakes
- Lunch: Beetroot and Ginger Soup
- Dinner: Grilled Swordfish with Salsa Verde
- Snack: Orange Gelatin

Sunday
- Breakfast: Avocado Smoothie
- Lunch: Mixed Greens with Apple Slices
- Dinner: Grilled Mackerel with Lime
- Snack: Fig Bars

Week 8

Monday
- Breakfast: Berry Banana Smoothie
- Lunch: Summer Corn Salad
- Dinner: Turkey Scallopini
- Snack: Oatmeal Cookies

Tuesday
- Breakfast: Pumpkin Spice Yogurt
- Lunch: Broccoli and Stilton Soup
- Dinner: Sautéed Shrimp with Ginger and Honey
- Snack: Tiramisu

Wednesday
- Breakfast: Ricotta and Pear Toast
- Lunch: Asian Vegetable Soup
- Dinner: Peppered Mackerel
- Snack: Almond Joy Bites

Thursday
- Breakfast: Cottage Cheese Pancakes
- Lunch: Carrot and Coriander Soup
- Dinner: Herbed Sea Bass
- Snack: Chocolate Covered Strawberries

Friday
- Breakfast: Almond Flour Pancakes
- Lunch: Leek and Potato Soup
- Dinner: Chili Lime Shrimp Skewers
- Snack: Vegetable Chips

Saturday
- Breakfast: Whole Wheat Toast
- Lunch: Cabbage Soup
- Dinner: Tandoori Chicken
- Snack: Cheese and Fruit Plate

Sunday
- Breakfast: Pineapple Coconut Smoothie
- Lunch: Beetroot and Ginger Soup
- Dinner: Thai Grilled Chicken
- Snack: Fig Bars

Week 9
Monday
- Breakfast: Buckwheat Pancakes
- Lunch: Spinach and Strawberry Salad
- Dinner: Grilled Clams with Garlic
- Snack: Orange Gelatin

Tuesday
- Breakfast: Mushroom and Spinach Sauté
- Lunch: Mixed Greens with Apple Slices
- Dinner: Baked Haddock with Tomatoes
- Snack: Frozen Yogurt Bark

Wednesday
- Breakfast: Quinoa Porridge
- Lunch: Summer Corn Salad
- Dinner: Lemon Pepper Catfish
- Snack: Baked Kale Chips

Thursday
- Breakfast: Avocado Smoothie
- Lunch: Waldorf Salad
- Dinner: Chicken Piccata
- Snack: Oatmeal Cookies

Friday
- Breakfast: Berry Banana Smoothie
- Lunch: Broccoli and Stilton Soup
- Dinner: Mustard Roasted Trout
- Snack: Chocolate Covered Strawberries

Saturday
- Breakfast: Cottage Cheese Pancakes
- Lunch: Mediterranean Chickpea Salad
- Dinner: Orange Glazed Halibut
- Snack: Vegetable Chips

Sunday
- Breakfast: Egg Muffins
- Lunch: Carrot and Coriander Soup
- Dinner: Grilled Sardines with Lemon
- Snack: Cheese and Fruit Plate

Week 10

Monday
- Breakfast: Pineapple Coconut Smoothie
- Lunch: Beetroot and Ginger Soup
- Dinner: Broiled Tilapia with Thyme
- Snack: Fig Bars

Tuesday
- Breakfast: Almond Flour Pancakes
- Lunch: Mixed Greens with Apple Slices
- Dinner: Spiced Roast Turkey
- Snack: Tiramisu

Wednesday
- Breakfast: Whole Wheat Toast
- Lunch: Broccoli and Stilton Soup
- Dinner: Grilled Tuna with Basil Pesto
- Snack: Frozen Yogurt Bark

Thursday
- Breakfast: Ricotta and Pear Toast
- Lunch: Asian Vegetable Soup
- Dinner: Pan-Seared Chicken with Spinach
- Snack: Orange Gelatin

Friday
- Breakfast: Cottage Cheese Pancakes
- Lunch: Summer Corn Salad
- Dinner: Herbed Sea Bass
- Snack: Baked Kale Chips

Saturday
- Breakfast: Quinoa Porridge
- Lunch: Cabbage Soup
- Dinner: Lemon Sole Meuniere
- Snack: Chocolate Covered Strawberries

Sunday
- Breakfast: Mushroom and Spinach Sauté
- Lunch: Spinach and Strawberry Salad
- Dinner: Chicken Marsala
- Snack: Vegetable Chips

WEEKLY MEAL PLANNER + WORKBOOK

	BREAKFAST	LUNCH	DINNER	SNACKS
MONDAY				
TUESDAY				
WEDNESDAY				
THURSDAY				
FRIDAY				
SATURDAY				
SUNDAY				

What are your current favorite meals, and how can you adapt them to be low sodium?

....

....

....

....

....

....

WEEKLY MEAL PLANNER + WORKBOOK

	BREAKFAST	LUNCH	DINNER	SNACKS
MONDAY				
TUESDAY				
WEDNESDAY				
THURSDAY				
FRIDAY				
SATURDAY				
SUNDAY				

What challenges do you anticipate facing while reducing sodium in your diet?

....

....

....

....

....

WEEKLY MEAL PLANNER + WORKBOOK

	BREAKFAST	LUNCH	DINNER	SNACKS
MONDAY				
TUESDAY				
WEDNESDAY				
THURSDAY				
FRIDAY				
SATURDAY				
SUNDAY				

List three herbs or spices you're excited to try as salt substitutes. Why do they appeal to you?

....

....

....

....

....

....

WEEKLY MEAL PLANNER + WORKBOOK

	BREAKFAST	LUNCH	DINNER	SNACKS
MONDAY				
TUESDAY				
WEDNESDAY				
THURSDAY				
FRIDAY				
SATURDAY				
SUNDAY				

Identify three high-sodium foods you commonly eat. What lower sodium alternatives could you try?

....

....

....

....

....

....

WEEKLY MEAL PLANNER + WORKBOOK

	BREAKFAST	LUNCH	DINNER	SNACKS
MONDAY				
TUESDAY				
WEDNESDAY				
THURSDAY				
FRIDAY				
SATURDAY				
SUNDAY				

What are some situations where you might find it difficult to stick to a low sodium diet? How will you handle them?

....

....

....

....

....

....

WEEKLY MEAL PLANNER + WORKBOOK

	BREAKFAST	LUNCH	DINNER	SNACKS
MONDAY				
TUESDAY				
WEDNESDAY				
THURSDAY				
FRIDAY				
SATURDAY				
SUNDAY				

Describe a recent meal you enjoyed. How might you modify it to fit a low sodium diet?

....

....

....

....

....

....

WEEKLY MEAL PLANNER + WORKBOOK

	BREAKFAST	LUNCH	DINNER	SNACKS
MONDAY				
TUESDAY				
WEDNESDAY				
THURSDAY				
FRIDAY				
SATURDAY				
SUNDAY				

What snacks do you typically reach for, and what are some low sodium options you could choose instead?

....

....

....

....

....

WEEKLY MEAL PLANNER + WORKBOOK

	BREAKFAST	LUNCH	DINNER	SNACKS
MONDAY				
TUESDAY				
WEDNESDAY				
THURSDAY				
FRIDAY				
SATURDAY				
SUNDAY				

What benefits do you hope to achieve by following a low sodium diet? List at least three.

....
....
....
....
....
....

WEEKLY MEAL PLANNER + WORKBOOK

	BREAKFAST	LUNCH	DINNER	SNACKS
MONDAY				
TUESDAY				
WEDNESDAY				
THURSDAY				
FRIDAY				
SATURDAY				
SUNDAY				

How do you plan to track your sodium intake? What tools or methods will you use?

....
....
....
....
....
....

WEEKLY MEAL PLANNER + WORKBOOK

	BREAKFAST	LUNCH	DINNER	SNACKS
MONDAY				
TUESDAY				
WEDNESDAY				
THURSDAY				
FRIDAY				
SATURDAY				
SUNDAY				

Think about dining out. What strategies can you use to ensure your meal remains low sodium?

....
....
....
....
....
....

WEEKLY MEAL PLANNER + WORKBOOK

	BREAKFAST	LUNCH	DINNER	SNACKS
MONDAY				
TUESDAY				
WEDNESDAY				
THURSDAY				
FRIDAY				
SATURDAY				
SUNDAY				

What are some low sodium foods you already enjoy? How can you incorporate more of them into your meals?

....

....

....

....

....

....

Scan the QR code below to get a surprise bonus!

www.ingramcontent.com/pod-product-compliance
Lightning Source LLC
Chambersburg PA
CBHW082235220526
45479CB00005B/1238